OVERCOMING LONELINESS

Overcoming Loneliness

Strategies for Finding
Joy and Building
Community

LESLIE PARKER TAYLOR
FOREWORD BY DANNY SILK

Overcoming Loneliness: Strategies for Finding Joy and Building Community by Leslie Taylor.

Copyright 2025 Leslie Taylor

All rights reserved. Printed in the United States of America.

No part of this publication may be reproduced or transmitted for commercial purposes, except for brief quotations in printed reviews, without written permission of the author.

Library of Congress Cataloging-in-Publication Data

ISBN: 979-8-89694-346-4 - Ebook

ISBN: 979-8-89694-347-1 - Paperback

ISBN: 979-8-89694-348-8 - Hardcover

Scripture quotations marked NIV are taken from the Holy Bible, New International Version®, NIV®. Copyright © 1973, 1978, 1984, 2011 by Biblica, Inc.™ Used by permission of Zondervan. All rights reserved worldwide. www.zondervan.com.

Scripture quotations marked NLT are taken from the Holy Bible, New Living Translation, copyright © 1996, 2004, 2015 by Tyndale House Foundation. Used by permission of Tyndale House Publishers, Inc., Carol Stream, Illinois 60188. All rights reserved.

Scriptures marked NKJV are taken from the New King James Version. Copyright© 1982 by Thomas Nelson, Inc. Used by permission. All rights reserved.

Scripture quotations marked TPT are from The Passion Translation®. Copyright © 2017, 2018, 2020 by Passion & Fire Ministries, Inc. Used by permission. All rights reserved. ThePassionTranslation.com.

The author has made every attempt to provide information that is accurate and complete, but this book is not intended as a substitute for professional medical advice or psychological therapy. This book is not meant to be used, nor should it be used, to diagnose or treat any medical or psychological condition.

First Edition: 2025

Note that names and details of individuals in some of the stories have been altered to protect their privacy.

This book is dedicated to my clients

ENDORSEMENTS

"As head of the Healing Ministry at Bethel for a number of years, I had the incredible privilege of working with Leslie and saw firsthand her dedication to those facing life's challenges, helping them find deep emotional healing. Her love for people and the depth of her knowledge and experience are outstanding, and she has done a fantastic job of capturing it in this book about the much-neglected topic of loneliness.

It's not just a how-to manual but a profound blending of personal wisdom from her own life experiences and those of people she has walked with. Somehow she has managed to give us all the how-tos without making them boring or condemning or just a list of more rules, instead making it all so straightforward, encouraging, and very possible. I'm honoured to give her work, both in person and in the pages of this book, my full endorsement. Read it and be blessed!"

Chris Gore
Chris Gore Ministries, New Zealand
Author of *How to Walk in Supernatural Healing Power, Apprehended Identity,*
and *#Positioned to Receive and Maintain Your Miracle*

"Leslie Taylor is one of the most gifted therapists I know. Her own personal journey plus her years of experience have given her so much wisdom and insight into how to truly help people. I'm really excited for this book, I know it's going to help so many people."

Jason Vallotton
Senior Leader, Bethel Church Redding
Founder of BraveCo
Author of several books, including *Winning the War Within: The Journey to Healing and Wholeness*, *The Supernatural Power of Forgiveness: Discover How to Escape Your Prison of Pain and Unlock a Life of Freedom*, and *Moral Revolution: The Naked Truth about Sexual Purity*.

"It is such an honor to be asked to endorse Leslie's new book, *Overcoming Loneliness*. I have watched Leslie tend to so many people's wounds either as the head of Bethel's Pastor On Call or more recently as a therapist at the Transformation Center. Community and building healthy connections is such a passion for Leslie. I love her heart for hurting people and believe this book will help you to overcome loneliness and walk in deeper connection with both people and God."

Dawna De Silva
Founder and co-leader of Bethel Sozo Ministry
Author of *Sozo: Saved, Healed, Delivered*; *Shifting Atmospheres*; *Overcoming Fear*; *Warring with Wisdom*; and *Prayers, Declarations, and Strategies*

"Leslie has hit a home run addressing the epidemic of loneliness, providing relevant and practical resources to help break the silence of suffering alone. Leslie's words of compassion and encouragement are an invitation to live the rich fullness of life God intended."

Yvonne Martinez
Bethel Transformation Center Ministries Coordinator
CADC-CS, ICCS, ICADC, NCAC-I, CRPS
Certified Clinical Trauma Professional-CCTP
Pastoral Sex Addiction Professional-PSAP
Author of 20 books, including *Dancing on the Graves of your Past*
and *Healing Trauma: Using Simplified Bethel Sozo Ministry*

"Loneliness is a pervasive problem in our world and an issue that we all struggle with at times. In this book, Leslie lets you know that you are not alone in your struggle and ambushes the lie that you feel lonely because something is wrong with you. More than that, she gives you practical strategies for dealing with the challenge of loneliness. Leslie is highly skilled in dealing with people, and the strategies contained in this book, I believe, will help you and your loved ones put an end to loneliness."

Janine Mason
Co-director of Heaven in Business
Author of *Dream Culture, Kingdom Tools for Teaching,* and *Hearing God at Work*

"What is wrong with me?"

"Nothing, my love. Welcome to being a human being."

TABLE OF CONTENTS

Foreword xix
Note from the Author xxi
Introduction: Why Write a Book on Loneliness? 1

Section 1
Situations: The Case for Loneliness

Introduction: Where is Everyone 57
Chapter 1: Loneliness Related to Relationship Dynamics 15
Personal Growth 17
Season of Life Dissonance 19
A Season of Introspection 21
Capacity 22
Introvert vs. Extrovert 22
Surface-Level vs. Deep Conversationalists 24
A Struggle with Lost Identity—Who Am I? What Is My Purpose? ... 25
Differences or Perception of Differences 26
The Lies We Believe 27
Facade 29
Secrets 30

Chapter 2: Loneliness Related to Personal Lifestyle Choices 33
New Sobriety 34
Moving 36
Demanding Job, Lack of Work-Life Balance 38
Traveling Job 38
Change of Job or Retirement 39
Living Remotely 39

Working Remotely 40
Lack of Income 41
Season of Life Requirements 41

Chapter 3: Loneliness Related to Extraordinary Circumstances 45

Caregiving 46
Illness or Lack of Mobility 47
Dietary and Other Accommodations 47
Mental Illness...47
Physical and Mental Disabilities..48
Abuse 48
Death of a Loved One..49
Divorce and Breakups 50
Traumatic Events and Disasters..51
The Pandemic Effect 52

Section 2
Solutions : What You Can Do to Be Proactive

Introduction: What to Do in the Meantime 57

1—Listen to How You Talk to Yourself 58
2—Take a Stance of Compassionate Curiosity 58
3—Acknowledge Your Feelings...59
4—Give Yourself Grace and Acceptance 60

Chapter 4: Becoming Your Own Best Friend 63

Practice Gratitude 65
Practice Being in the Present with Mindfulness..................67
Reset Your Vagus Nerve..68
Take a Break...69
Laugh...71
Challenge Your Negative Thoughts 72
Get Outdoors...74
Get Moving..76
Practice Self-Care 76

Get Healthy 78
Work on Personal Growth and Self-Reflection 79
Connect to Your Heart 80
Pursue Creativity 82
Start a Collection 83
Engage in Hobbies 84
Give Attention to Your Home and Yard 85
Get That "Other" To-Do List Done 86
Learn a New Musical Instrument or Language 88
Learn a New Tech-Related Skill 88
Travel 89
Adopt a Pet 90
Make a New Friend-Connect with a Professional Listening Service .. 93
Seek Professional Support 94

Chapter 5: Connecting with Others 97

Reconnect with People from Your Past on Social Media 100
Write Handwritten Letters and Cards 101
Reinvest in Groups You Are Already In 102
Engage More Deeply with Co-Workers 103
Explore Online Communities that Share a Similar Interest 105
Join a Local Support Group 106
Meet with Others Who Share Your Passion 107
Take a Class in the Community 108
Join an Exercise Group 109
Become a Community Volunteer 110
Elevate Your Social Skills 111
Start a Home Group 112
Be Proactive 113

Section 3
Considerations: How to Optimize and Not Sabotage Yourself

Introduction: A Few Things to Consider 119

Chapter 6: Self-Sabotaging Coping Behaviors 121

Substance Abuse 123
Excessive Shopping 125
Pornography 126
Poor Self-Care 127
Isolation 128
Me-Focus 128
The Blame Game 129
Negative Thoughts 130
Losing Hope 131
Depression 132

Chapter 7:   Taking Personal Inventory 137

Egocentrism 138
Talking a Lot 140
Oversharing 141
Always Shallow 142
Not a Great Listener 143
No Eye Contact 144
Distracted 145
Interrupting 146
Advice-Giving 147
Boring 148
Poor Hygiene 149
Always Accepting, Never Inviting 150
Never Offering Use of Your Home or Car 150
Expecting Others to Always Work Around Your Schedule 151
Gossipy 152
Being Negative/Critical 153

Chapter 8:   When to Seek Help 157

Severe Depression 158
Self-Imposed Extreme Isolation 160
Debilitating Anxiety 160
A Persistent Feeling of Loneliness All of One's Life 161
Intrusive Thoughts or Repetitive Behaviors 162
Driven by Only What Benefits You 163

Deep Despair, Suicidal Thoughts 163

Section 4
Loved Ones: Helping Those You Love Thrive

Introduction: When You Are Concerned for
Someone Else 169

Chapter 9: How to Help Your Lonely Child 171
Be Available 174
Be Nonjudgmental 175
Teach Your Child How to Manage Their Inner Dialogue 176
Teach Your Child Values 177
Teach Your Child Good Social Skills 178
Teach Your Child How to Be a Good Friend 179
Facilitate Friendships 180
Help Your Child Develop into an Interesting Person 181
Volunteer Together 183
Seek Professional Support 184

Chapter 10: How to Help Your Lonely Aging Parents .. 187
Watch Television Together 191
Do Jigsaw Puzzles Together 191
Get Them a Pet 191
Help with Social Media 192
Go on Field Trips 192
Send Cards and Letters 193
Engage Delivery Services 193
Hire Help 194
Watch Shows, Documentaries, and Movies Apart but Together 195
Make Phone Calls and Video Calls 195
Assemble and Send an Activity Box 196
Help Your Parent Get Connected in the Community 196
Help Them Find Purpose and Fulfillment 197
Encourage Them to Explore New Interests 198
Hire a Professional Listening Service 199

The Conclusion and More

Conclusion: Is This Forever?. 203
Final Thoughts from My Heart 205
Next Steps. 211
And … How You Can Help! 213
Resources 215
Acknowledgments 217
About the Author 223

FOREWORD

The book you're holding is written by someone I know and trust, a person who is skilled and talented in meeting people where they are and helping them find solutions. I believe this book is going to be a supportive resource to so many who are battling the fog of loneliness.

I remember reading, "I was on the verge of total ruin, in the midst of the assembly and congregation" (Proverbs 5:14 NKJV), and it shocked me to realize we can indeed be so alone in the midst of a crowd. We can go to church, the office, school, or a family reunion and still leave feeling disconnected. Often, no one notices we are living with an ongoing experience of isolation and painful separation. But why? Why are we so alone?

It is easier than ever to have this experience. Our present society is almost making it a goal to be alone while watching others live life. Technology feeds us what we want to see, tells us what we want to hear, and entertains us with what we want, encouraging us to become spectators. This seems like a dangerous path for mankind.

Building and maintaining strong, healthy connections with other human beings is not easy. On the other hand, experiencing offense or disconnection with humans is very easy. Navigating the course of finding, strengthening, and healing relationships requires a committed journey.

Please allow Leslie Taylor to come alongside you and support you while you take this journey. Right away, you won't be alone because Leslie will have your hand. I understand it takes great courage to hope for a breakthrough, but please take this next little while to let someone help you see the light at the end of the tunnel.

God Bless,

Danny Silk
Founder of Loving on Purpose
Author of *Keep Your Love On*

NOTE FROM THE AUTHOR

Welcome to a practical guide on navigating a season of loneliness. I hope it blesses you.

Stories in this book are based on real situations I've experienced, and others have been experienced by my family, friends, and clients. In most cases, names and identifying information have been changed to protect privacy. In some cases, the stories of several people have been combined to incorporate the experiences of more people. A few friends gave me permission to use their real names.

Some chapters contain lists of suggestions. You may notice some ideas on these lists are repeated in several places throughout the book. This is done purposefully so that the reader can flip to whatever section fits their situation best and not miss out on ideas that might benefit them. While there is a lot of information and encouragement unique to each chapter woven throughout the book that I believe can benefit the reader no matter their situation, I realize that sometimes you want to just get to the part that fits you.

Additionally, I know there are a lot of deep and complicated issues involved in loneliness. I want to acknowledge that this will not be a deep dive into the scientific research on loneliness or the social issues of our times that can separate people and contribute to loneliness. And though I am a Christian therapist and write from that perspective, I will not be delving into the deeper spiritual issues that can accompany loneliness either. A book could be written on each of these topics alone. The focus of this book is intentionally meant to be narrower and more on practical application. I openly share some of my personal encounters with the Lord in these pages, but my experience does not have to be your experience. Wherever you are in your experience of God and life, it is my hope that this book will be useful to you and bless your life.

INTRODUCTION

WHY WRITE A BOOK ON LONELINESS?

Sitting with someone behind a closed door as they share their deepest thoughts and feelings is a deep honor. It is a sacred space. It is the space I am called to.

It is in that sacred space that I have found client after client so vulnerably sharing how lonely they are. It is the rare client that doesn't express that feeling at some point. Additionally, most of my clients are struggling with the thought, *Is something wrong with me?* The discouragement is high. The struggle is real.

My clients span all ages, both men and women, in a variety of professions, with differing cultures, personalities, experiences, and levels of emotional and spiritual maturity, influence, economic status, and renown. And yet across the board, so many of them have this one thing in common—loneliness.

I really love my clients. It's impossible to get to know someone on an intimate heart level and not love them. And I believe their experience speaks to the experience of many others. If you are struggling with loneliness, know that you are not alone. There is hope!

Let me introduce myself. I am a therapist at the Bethel Transformation Center in Redding, California. I am also an entrepreneur. Writing this book sort of encompasses both worlds. My journey in this direction officially started when I went back to college to complete my bachelor's and pursue a master's degree in marriage and family therapy after my three kids started school. It took a few years, and in the process, I became a single mom. When my fifteen-year-old daughter died a few years after I established my private practice, I found myself needing a new direction. From there, I went on to what I later came to recognize as an extraordinary "experience collecting" journey. I married my wonderful husband, Tom, in 1999.

Now I'm back full circle, working as a therapist in a church setting with a few decades of experience as a police officer, crisis pastor, public speaker, businesswoman, and disaster worker under my belt. All those experiences, combined with a number of life-altering experiences and a deep faith and love for the Lord, have forever shaped me. I'd like to call myself just a wise older woman, but that sounds a little presumptuous—and old. If I had to label what I do at the Transformation

Center, I would say I am a pastoral therapist. Sometimes my role may also include being a mentor, a consultant, a coach, or even simply a mom or a sister in Christ.

Back to our topic …

One doesn't have to look very far to realize loneliness could qualify as an epidemic in our society—especially since the COVID-19 pandemic of 2020, when so many of us were shut in our homes for an extended period of time. A 2020 study by AARP showed two-thirds of American adults were experiencing loneliness and increased anxiety during that time. Interestingly, a Cigna report revealed greater levels of loneliness were experienced by millennials and Generation Z in 2020 than by older adults. Having witnessed the mental decline of many older adults during that time, it is hard for me to imagine. But considering the greater level of social activity this younger age group is used to, it does make sense.

On top of that, nearly half of all adults in the United States were still feeling a negative impact a year later! A post-pandemic survey conducted by the Kaiser Family Foundation in 2021 found that 47 percent of American adults felt their mental health was negatively impacted by the isolation experienced during the pandemic. Social dynamics changed dramatically, and we are still adjusting.

We can't blame it all on the pandemic of 2020, though. Loneliness has been an issue for a long time; it was only exacerbated by the pandemic. Look at these numbers:

- 2010 – One-third of the adults in the US over age forty-five reported being lonely. (*Time* magazine)
- 2017 – Vivek Murthy, the US Surgeon General, called loneliness a growing health epidemic in the US.
- 2018 – One in three older adults in the US reported struggling with loneliness (56 percent reported in 2020, University of Michigan).

The issue is not just in the United States, either. Loneliness is a worldwide concern:

- 2018 – UK Prime Minister Theresa May appointed Tracey Crouch as the country's first Minister for Loneliness, two years after creating a commission on loneliness.
- 2022 – A report by Michael Vecchio (*World Atlas*, December 2022) ranked the top ten countries for loneliness. Sweden was at the top of the list, with 47 percent of the population reporting feelings of loneliness, followed by the UK, Japan, Italy, the US, Canada, Russia, South Africa, Kenya, and Brazil—in that order.

There are health implications as well:

- 2023 – The World Health Organization (WHO) declared loneliness a "global health threat."
- 2023 – The US Surgeon General compared the health consequences of loneliness to that of smoking fifteen cigarettes a day.
- The negative effects from loneliness have been found to be more harmful than obesity, alcoholism, or a lack of physical activity. An increased risk of heart disease, stroke, lowered immunity, cognitive decline, mental illness, depression, suicide, and premature death by as much as fifteen years have all been associated with loneliness.

Outcomes aside, the experience of loneliness in and of itself can be excruciatingly painful and usually plays into overall discouragement about life.

Because of these conversations with clients and friends behind closed doors and because of the bigger picture, including the impact loneliness has had on our society, I decided to write this book. I want you to know that you are not alone, and this does not have to be your permanent lot in life. There is a way out!

This book is divided into four main sections, followed by a fifth concluding section:

- **Section 1** will focus on why loneliness is so pervasive, looking at relationship dynamics, choices we make, and extraordinary circumstances. Understanding the why behind your struggle with loneliness can be validating, but it doesn't solve the problem, so ...
- **Section 2** focuses on solutions, looking at practical things you can do, both alone and in building relationships.
- **Section 3** will talk about cautions—temptations to watch out for and personal habits that might benefit from an upgrade in order to help you forge connections with others. (The last chapter in Section 3 addresses when it might be important to get professional help.)
- **Section 4** discusses the topic of helping those you love who may be lonely, specifically addressing children and elderly parents.
- **The Conclusion and More** includes the Conclusion (of course), plus Final Thoughts from My Heart, Resources, Acknowledgements, About the Author, and Next Steps.

Woven throughout the chapters in this book are these truths I really want you to know:

- If you feel lonely, you are not alone.
- You are not a fatally flawed human being.
- Loneliness is temporary.
- With proactive, persistent work, you can emerge and even flourish!

I have written this book with my clients and all who are lonely and hurting throughout the world in mind. If that includes you, my hope above all is that you will feel seen and understood. In addition to that, I hope you also feel encouraged and maybe even a little more empowered by what you find within the pages of this book. Happy reading!

A WORD OF ENCOURAGEMENT

If you are struggling with loneliness, there is nothing wrong with you. It is a global epidemic. But take heart! Loneliness does not have to swallow up your entire life. I have no doubt that you, like many others, can emerge from loneliness by implementing some of the mindsets and strategies shared in this book.

If you are not struggling with loneliness but love someone who is, thank you for caring for them so deeply. May this book give you just what you need to offer them hope and encouragement.

SECTION 1

SITUATIONS

THE CASE FOR LONELINESS

SECTION 1 INTRODUCTION

WHERE IS EVERYONE?

Causes of Loneliness

There are many different reasons people are lonely. It can be very simple to sort out in some situations, but it can also be quite complex at times, with multiple reasons factoring in. It is interesting to me that my clients rarely appear to have any glaring characteristics or behaviors that seem to be the cause. Even when clients show up convinced there is something wrong with them and share everything they think might be the reason for their loneliness, I've found little evidence to support the idea that they are socially undesirable. You can garner a small amount of comfort in looking around and seeing that there is a tribe to fit almost every "awkward" person you know. Being a perfect human being does not seem to be a requirement for winning friends and combating loneliness.

If you are currently beating yourself up and wondering what is wrong with you, please know it is about what is happening in the world. Despite all the ways we can connect through technology, we are so much more disconnected from friends and family compared to fifty years ago.

In this section, I have listed out all the factors that I repeatedly see contributing to the loneliness people are experiencing and divided them into the following three categories:

- Chapter 1: Loneliness Related to Relationship Dynamics
- Chapter 2: Loneliness Related to Lifestyle Choices
- Chapter 3: Loneliness Related to Extraordinary Circumstances

These categories are admittedly imperfect and overlap, but they will work for our purposes.

My hope is that you will have some *aha moments* as you read through this section and maybe come to some further understanding of why you or someone you love is feeling so lonely. Some of these reasons are obvious, and I can see the reader going, "Duh," as they read them. I'm okay with that. My purpose is to hopefully bring to your mind some new realizations about how different factors may be contributing to this struggle with loneliness. Some of these involve the person who is feeling lonely, but it more often includes a much bigger picture. There are many reasons why so many people are struggling with loneliness in our world, and understanding this can boost morale and obliterate that sense of shame that so often accompanies loneliness.

If you are still convinced that something lacking in yourself is the cause of your loneliness, you can jump ahead to Chapter 7 and do a self-inventory of sorts. The traits covered in Chapter 7 are traits most of us can improve upon. If nothing else, maybe that chapter will stand alone as a good personal checklist for anyone seeking to be a more thoughtful human being in social settings.

So, what is causing us as a world population to be so lonely? Let's start by looking at loneliness related to relationship dynamics.

CHAPTER 1

LONELINESS RELATED TO RELATIONSHIP DYNAMICS

It is my belief that feelings of abandonment and rejection create possibly the deepest experience of emotional pain we as humans can feel. They are feelings that I witness go even deeper than the grief experienced in the loss of a loved one. I believe this is because the death of another person happens outside of us, whereas abandonment and rejection go to the core of our very being and evoke questions about our self-worth.

My point is not to minimize the pain of grief. That pain is real and is hopefully well validated in later pages in this book. The point I want to make here is that we all need to feel seen and heard, understood and valued, yet it is not an uncommon experience to feel invisible and alone. It is not unusual to wrestle with the pain of abandonment and rejection.

We are created to belong, to be surrounded by people who see us, understand us, love us, and care for us. We are created to provide that sense of belonging to others as well. When that need to be a part of a family or friendship community is unmet or thwarted, there is real pain. That pain runs underneath everything else we might do. It may be experienced in a loud and screaming way, demanding attention, or it may be more of a quiet sadness, pressed down, buried deep within the secret caverns of the soul.

Loneliness, at its core, is rooted in the absence of relationships that the heart longs for. But herein lies the challenge—relationships are not a solitary venture. Other people are involved, and this adds complexity. Though all the chapters in this section somewhat overlap, in this first chapter, we will look at matters of the heart, factors involved in relationship dynamics that can cause dissonance and lead a person to feel disconnected and lonely. In Chapters 2 and 3, we will focus more on the external relationship factors that can come into play in loneliness.

Relationships are complicated. If they weren't problematic, I'd be out of a job. Each of us brings our own unique history and personality into a relationship. And though there are arguably exceptions, most people are also growing and changing with time, adding to the complication. We come to whatever stage we are in life armed with our experiences and what we have deduced about life from those experiences, and without exception, we tend to come with baggage and wounds as well. Some wounds have healed, and we have the scars to prove it. Other wounds are still in process and may be open, gaping, and painful. We come with beliefs, opinions, knowledge, and experiences that have either made us better or worse human beings. The differences we experience in each other are a part of our uniqueness; they can be attractive and add to the spark of connection, or they can cause separation and pain and be difficult to navigate.

Let's look at some of those possible pain points leading to loneliness. Determining what is underneath the disconnection cannot only bring understanding, but it can also help you come up with solutions for either shortening the season or making the best of it.

Personal Growth

April's husband, Ken, confessed to her that he had recently ended a year-long affair. His desire to get his life in line with his core values included being honest with his wife. The resulting confession was a complete surprise to April and threw their marriage, understandably, into crisis. They knew they needed help and quickly sought help from their church leaders, whom they found to be supportive and in agreement that Ken needed to step down from his ministry position for the time being. All agreed the couple needed to get into counseling, and it was the consensus of everyone that they should start with individual therapy. April became a client of mine about a month after her husband's confession.

As Ken and April worked through the individual issues they both felt had contributed, as well as all of the resulting issues that came up from such a break in trust, they were able to heal their marriage. Not a lot of couples can do this without also being in couples counseling, but they were able to do so. They both jumped on the opportunity to forgive, recommit, rebuild trust, and grow.

While doing so, they started recognizing unhealthy patterns in their friends and family. As they were learning to face hard issues, set healthy boundaries, and have difficult conversations in which they chose to be honest and vulnerable, their friends and even some family members distanced themselves. They found themselves feeling less connected to friends and acquaintances who tended to play games of avoidance, manipulation, gaslighting, and passive aggressiveness instead of expressing what they were feeling in real and honest conversation. In that place of deep personal growth, they found themselves feeling more and more alone.

As people progress on their own personal growth journeys, they often start seeing behaviors in their friends that they no longer tolerate in themselves. It gets harder and harder to maintain close friendships with people who are still stuck in behaviors that they now recognize as unhealthy. Developing new friendships that are healthier can take time, often leaving a person with a "gap" in friends.

This is the number one reason my clients are experiencing loneliness, and that makes sense. People who go to counseling are typically people who are looking to grow and become healthier human beings. When I share that this "friend gap" is a normal progression seen commonly in personal growth journeys, it generally resonates with them. They just didn't know it was a "thing."

> NOTE: It is super important to partner with God in loving your old friends well—not picking up any unforgiveness or offense. There is no room for arrogance or disdain, though that is sometimes the natural temptation. It's healthy to allow friends to be where they are in their own life journey. You may simply need to set a different boundary with them now. Treasure who they have been in your lives. Treat them well. Everyone has their own timetable and different desires about who they want to be, as well as possibly even different beliefs about what their possibilities for change are. Know that as you get healthier, you will start attracting healthier people to you. It can take time, but it happens. Use this time to truly pursue the heart of God.

Season of Life Dissonance

Judy is a client of mine in her mid-forties. All her life, she has wanted to get married and have a family. She continued to believe it would happen for her, and throughout her twenties and thirties, she celebrated with friends who saw their dreams coming true, attending their weddings and baby showers. She was truly happy for them. But eventually, the reality of her age started setting in, and she realized, short of a miracle, she was not going to be able to have her own biological babies.

Many of my single clients struggle with watching their friends progress into a season of marriage and family. They may feel a loss as their best girlfriend or guy friend starts focusing their time and attention in another direction. It can become overwhelming for single individuals over time as more and more of their friends step into these life transitions. At some point, they may look around and feel left behind.

The pain of not finding your soulmate or not having a family of your own can be crushing. Often, the belief that something must be wrong with you adds to the pain. As if that weren't enough, feeling like you are losing your friends can cause almost unbearable feelings of loneliness, as they step into their dreams while yours go unfulfilled.

If you find yourself in a similar situation, allow yourself to grieve. Shifts in your friendship circles are real losses. Grieve your loss, care for your heart, and then find your new tribe. You will find them. Don't give up. Hopefully, you will find some ideas for how to do so in this book.

A Season of Introspection

Another time I see people struggling with loneliness is when they are feeling somewhat overwhelmed with disappointment about their life, and that feeling pulls them inward. There are plenty of people who have a natural tendency toward introspection. They like to process things alone first before talking to a friend. That is not what I am talking about here. That is more situational and short-term.

Where introspection connects with loneliness is when a person feels they can't talk with anyone about something going on in their life, so all of their processing about it is done internally, alone. They may be embarrassed or ashamed about how they feel, or they may be driven by the need to protect another person's privacy. Sometimes, working through things alone comes from the belief that no one would understand. This belief can make a person feel deeply alone.

Some of the disappointments I have seen affecting people in this way include discouragement about not being married or great sadness about the state of their marriage; feelings of inadequacy as a parent, or maybe not even enjoying parenthood; struggles with fertility; challenges with adult children or emotionally unhealthy parents; job burnout or feeling trapped in a career path they have come to hate; struggles with friends; and concerns about money. Any of these can create the feeling of being alone, even if one is surrounded by friends.

Capacity

The season of life a person is in may limit their capacity for social activities, no matter how much they would like to engage. Beth, a client of mine, has five young children. Her life keeps her busy, and by evening time, when her church offers women's activities she could join, she finds she is too tired and has no capacity to socialize—despite her loneliness and her husband's offer to babysit. This is a common problem.

Other factors can play a part in limiting the energy or capacity you have available for making new friends. These may include the demands of a job or business, demands of balancing both a family and a job, special needs within your family, health challenges, sleep challenges, the needs of extended family, discouragement, depression, or being overwhelmed. Many times, like with my client Beth, a limited capacity is the very thing that makes it difficult to create social options that work for you.

Introvert vs. Extrovert

Introversion and extroversion are personality traits that fall on a continuum. Extroverts tend to process information externally and with others. Additionally, they get energy from social interaction. Introverts tend to be quieter and process information internally; they may enjoy being social, but typically, social interactions drain their energy. They recharge by being alone. (Ambiverts tend to fall in the middle, being a mix of the two.)

Extreme introversion can create an aversion to social events, which can contribute to the experience of loneliness. Not only may there be a preference for quiet, which inhibits the desire to get out and mingle with others, but these traits also often correlate with a feeling of being socially awkward, which makes the aversion to socializing even greater. During the pandemic, many extroverts were feeling a great amount of stress being sequestered in their homes, whereas more introverted people reported enjoying the quiet opportunity to unplug and hibernate for a while.

In my practice, I have witnessed a very interesting dynamic in this regard. My more introverted clients have found it much harder to get out and reestablish the social connections they had pre-pandemic. They are even struggling with the effort required to respond to the invitations of others—while simultaneously grieving the lack of connection with friends. What took a long time to establish now feels overwhelming to reestablish.

Meanwhile, my more extroverted clients have reported frustration at their perceived inability to get their more introverted friends to "come out and play" for the same reason. There is no right or wrong here. I've witnessed both personality types feeling the effects of the pandemic and struggling to reconnect.

Additionally, when one person has less need for frequent connection, the relationship can become imbalanced, as the burden to connect always falls on the one wanting it more. This imbalance can get old for the one who must always do the instigating, and it is not unusual to see their desire to connect wane over time.

Everyone needs to feel that their friendship is valued. When the initiation for connection always falls on one person, it is easy to feel like the other person doesn't really care about having a relationship. From my experience with clients, the introvert/extrovert dynamic commonly plays a part in the loneliness people are experiencing.

Surface-Level vs. Deep Conversationalists

A common complaint my clients bring into the office is that they can't find anyone willing to have a deep, meaningful conversation that goes beyond just surface-level talk. Sometimes, it is an issue of difference of desires, but sometimes, it is an issue of timing. Connection can be affected either way. The person who longs for deeper, meaningful conversation can feel hesitant to pursue a relationship with someone who never goes below surface-level, while a person who reserves deeper conversations for only their very closest friends or family members may feel uncomfortable and back away from getting to know someone who wants to talk on a deeper level too soon.

Client after client tells me they long for deeper, meaningful conversations with people. I often wish I could introduce my clients to one another. I think they would like each other! The number of clients I have who express this desire far outnumber the clients who want conversations to stay surface-level. Then again, the latter are probably not the ones who find the thought of counseling appealing!

From my observation, there is no shortage of people who prefer surface-level conversation. It's the ones who long for more in-depth connection in their friendships who are struggling with loneliness, challenged to find people like themselves.

A Struggle with Lost Identity—Who Am I? What Is My Purpose?

I live in a culture where purpose, dreams, vision, achievement, and goals are topics talked about almost daily. Maybe it is the culture of America. If you operate in the business realm, it is a common topic, but it can be found anywhere—in education, in the arts, in churches. It is pretty much everywhere. As common as these topics are, it is also common for a person to wrestle with what their purpose is, what they were created for—what their legacy will be—to the point of real frustration.

When people do not have a strong sense of identity, when they do not feel like they know who they are—especially when they feel like everyone else does—it causes them to feel very lonely. I see this a lot with my clients who have given their entire lives to raising their family and have since seen their kids leave home. I also see it with clients coming out of long-term emotionally abusive relationships. Barbara, a brand-new client, said in her initial session, "I don't even know what I like anymore. I don't know what my favorite color is or even my favorite food. I lost myself somewhere along the way." I hear this all the time.

Maybe one of the loneliest feelings is when you feel like you've lost yourself.

Differences or Perception of Differences

While smaller communities frequently offer an advantage in the way of feeling known and creating that sense of connection and belonging, they can also present a greater challenge if that smaller community is made up of people who are different from you. For whatever reason, you just don't jibe naturally—but all you have is each other, so you make the best of it.

Having different interests can make it hard to find common ground for building a relationship with someone. Even if two people or a group of people have a common interest, it is not uncommon to find that schedules are incompatible, making it difficult to find a common available time to connect.

Differences can be real, but they can also be pure perception. Whether real or perceived, these differences can lead people to believe they haven't truly found their tribe yet, they don't connect easily with anyone around them, or they haven't met anyone they *want* to connect with. This can serve to further isolate people and contribute to loneliness. The options in a small town are more limited and can lead one to believe it will always be this way.

The Lies We Believe

We believe so many lies. Some come from others, and some we create in our own minds. Either way, it is a challenge to discover them and root them out.

I struggled with feeling tired for a full year and basically lost the entire year to it, going to work, coming home, and crashing. Then one day, I was crawling out of the driver's side of my car in our garage. I remember hearing myself sigh and thinking, *I'm so tired.* Just then, I heard the Lord say very clearly within my head, "You're not tired!"

My instant reply, admittedly very sarcastic and irreverent, was "Hmph, *okay*! I'm *not* tired!" Not one ounce of me believed that. But the moment I said, "I'm not tired," even in disbelief, I immediately felt energized and not tired at all. It was a dramatic shift. Maybe you can imagine my shock. Then He said to me, "My people are prisoners in their own minds." His point was made. I'd been a prisoner in my own mind, my body even bowing to the lie, and I'd lost a whole year of productivity because of it. The tiredness left and my energy returned when I broke my agreement with the lie.

> NOTE: I am not saying all tiredness is a lie. If you are tired, it is a good idea to get checked out by a doctor. This is just an example of my situation, when it was a lie, and my believing it affected my life significantly. The bigger point is that we have lies we believe that hold us prisoner. What lies might you be believing?

Bryan, a client of mine, made it clear to me that he was seeing me for one appointment and one appointment only. He just had one burning question he wanted to ask. He needed to know if something he was experiencing in his thought life was weird. He told me about it, and I assured him it was not. It's not unusual to have clients come to me just to find out if they are weird or if something is wrong with them.

The lies we believe can keep us isolated. We may believe the lie that we will be rejected when, in reality, we might find acceptance. We might have ourselves convinced that no one will believe us when they actually will. This, then, can result in separation and prolonged loneliness.

> NOTE: For an insightful and fascinating read on what believing lies looks like in the spirit realm, I highly recommend Blake K. Healy's book *Indestructible*.

Facade

My twenty-one-year-old cousin-in-law hung himself in our barn when I was a teenager. He had the biggest smile of anyone I knew. A friend who had seen him and stopped to chat with him minutes before had no idea what he was headed to do. He gave no indication. This, sadly, was the beginning of my understanding of how many sad people put on a happy face for the world. Sadder still is that we are often taught to do that ourselves.

Sometimes, a person can hold such a perfectionistic standard of what they want people to believe about them that they can't relax, let down their guard, and be themselves. The need to create a facade in which vulnerability and transparency are not a part of the relationship makes it hard to feel "at home" in a relationship because you cannot be yourself.

I can't imagine how lonely my cousin must have felt, keeping up the facade in front of all his friends. His case might seem like an extreme example, but I know it wasn't isolated. When a person doesn't or can't let down their guard and be themselves, connection becomes challenging because it cannot be authentic. If my cousin had been able to share his pain, I like to believe he would have found there was nothing wrong with him, that he was not alone. With half a chance, perhaps someone could have helped him walk out of that season into a brighter one.

Secrets

Sometimes, a person is harboring a secret that feels unsafe to share with anyone else. My client Robin was looking for a safe place to talk about challenges in her marriage. She was in leadership at a church and didn't feel it was safe to talk with anyone for fear it would bring judgment and affect her influence. All of her friends were connected to her church, leaving her feeling she had no one she could confide in. She felt very alone.

I live in a place where there are many highly gifted prophetic people, feelers, and seers in the spirit realm. It is not an uncommon experience to feel like someone just "read your mail." For someone who is hiding something, it can be an unsettling and even threatening environment. Whether in a highly prophetic environment or not, having a secret to protect can cause a person to self-isolate—to protect that secret from being found out—and this can lead to loneliness.

Sometimes, the challenge in a relationship is due to another person's life changing.

For example, if you are in a relationship with someone who has become isolated because of certain factors in their life, you can also experience the loss of the connection you once had with this person and feel loneliness because *their* circumstances are changing.

A WORD OF ENCOURAGEMENT

My purpose is to hopefully bring to your mind some new realizations about how different factors may be contributing to your struggle with loneliness. Life is complicated. Relationships are complicated. Having a personal relationship with God can help mitigate the pain of loneliness, but He created us to be in relationships with others also, so desiring connection is normal and a vital part of how you were created. (For more about a personal relationship with God, see Final Thoughts from My Heart and the Resources page, included in the Conclusion section of this book.)

This chapter hopefully gave you some helpful insights into how relationship dissonance contributes to loneliness. You may have already identified the factors that affect your own relationships, but there can still be great value in finding clarity and recognizing it is not all on you. Next, let's look at how lifestyle choices can impact loneliness.

CHAPTER 2

LONELINESS RELATED TO PERSONAL LIFESTYLE CHOICES

In the last chapter, we looked at factors within relationships that can cause dissonance, contributing to disconnection and loneliness—including decisions made by others that can impact us. In this chapter, we will look at how personal lifestyle choices can impact loneliness.

It's important to realize that the decisions we make in our lives may be responsible for throwing us into a season of loneliness. Sometimes, these decisions need to be made—they are choices made to better one's life. It's just that they often come with relationship price tags. Identifying how those lifestyle choices have negatively impacted you may help facilitate the decision to do something different.

For example, I have a client who is a traveling nurse. She has come to recognize that while her job is well-paying, the travel involved in her career is causing a lack of community in her life—and she has come to a time in her life when she wants to have community. She would like to get out of nursing altogether, but she wants to buy a house, so finances dictate that she stay in the profession for now. Consequently, she is looking for a nursing position she could enjoy that doesn't involve travel.

This kind of awareness brings clarity and, subsequently, the ability to weigh the costs versus the benefits. Increased awareness leads to opportunities to examine what we can change, and it empowers us to either make a change or make peace with our current circumstances if the cost is too great or they cannot be changed. Increasing your understanding of the "whys" contributing to your personal experience of loneliness can help you lead a more intentional life, helping you create the life you want.

Here are some examples of how one's personal lifestyle choices can spur a season of loneliness (you may be able to think of more):

New Sobriety

I met Garrett in a Christian singles group. He was a brand-new Christian. We became fast friends. When we lost the organizers of our singles group after one organizational meeting, I picked up the reins and started coordinating all our singles events. At that time, I was a police officer and had previously been in private practice as a therapist, so I was very familiar with addictions. Being in charge of the events, I took a hard "no alcohol" stance because I didn't want any of our gatherings to bring temptation to someone who might be struggling with sobriety. I wanted it to be a safe place for everyone.

A few months into our newly formed group, Garrett shared with me that he was a Friday-night-after-work beer drinker with the guys from work. He said that he always found himself drinking more on those Friday night occasions than he planned. Because of this, he decided he wanted to stop drinking altogether and felt I was a good friend to keep him accountable.

Truth is, I never had to say a word. He stopped drinking then and there. What I remember, as our friendship grew, was that he found himself no longer comfortable hanging out with his old friends because they all drank whenever they got together.

The timing of our singles group was good for him. He was already making new friends and was fortunate in that he was spared the lonely in-between season so many people face when they decide to give up drinking, drugs, or other unhealthy behaviors they have shared with friends. The connection shared with friends engaging in those behaviors is no longer there, and those relationships can even be an impediment to living differently. I see clients facing this issue too. Typically, there is a gap in friendships until new ones are made. It can be a tough and lonely season.

Moving

Moving usually entails starting your life all over again—a lot of new beginnings. Some moves will be less traumatic than others, but every move involves some level of change, and sometimes that change can be incredibly stressful. This is true whether you are moving to an entirely new state or country, moving back to a community where you previously lived, leaving home to go to college, or even just moving to a new neighborhood in the same city.

When we bought our first "starter home" in a brand-new subdivision, everyone in the neighborhood was a new homeowner. Almost every home had small children, and no one had fences yet. The kids freely ran through the backyards and in and out of each other's homes. The kids were the glue that brought the adults together, and friendships followed. It was a great neighborhood—even after everyone got fences.

A few years later, we were able to "upgrade" and move into a beautiful subdivision where the homes were twice as expensive as our prior neighborhood. We were so excited about our new home and neighborhood. That excitement quickly turned to disappointment as I found myself being snubbed by my new neighbors. I didn't understand the cold response. Someone finally explained to me that the prior owners of our house had divorced after the wife caught her husband cheating on her—and everyone had been friends with them, so the whole neighborhood was hurting. Apparently, my moving into "her" house added me to the list of wrongs done to her. On top of that, my kids were bullied by boys who lived down the street, and my next-door neighbor made it very clear to me that she didn't like children and wanted me to keep my kids away.

For a while, I was convinced that we were a family who fit in better with lower-income families. Fortunately, over time, the bullying stopped, and once my neighbors (with the exception of the one next door) got to know me for who I was, we became friends. But it was always a very different neighborhood from our first, and friendships from the first neighborhood have carried over even to this day.

Some neighborhoods are very friendly, and a lot of effort is made to welcome new neighbors. Others are more transient and less connected. You may find yourself in a neighborhood where no one seems to care that you are new and where everyone tends to live their own life apart from their neighbors. If you move to a neighborhood like this or even land in one where you don't really identify or "click" with the people who live around you, it can be hard to make friends. In such cases, it can feel pretty lonely—especially if your prior neighborhood was friendly and you felt known there.

Demanding Job, Lack of Work-Life Balance

Sometimes, a career can demand so much of a person's time that they don't have the time available to develop relationships. I could share example after example of clients who come into my office talking about how their dad worked all the time when they were growing up. They knew their dad was showing his love for his family by providing for them, but they missed having a nurturing relationship with that parent. It was not uncommon for their mom to be busy with household responsibilities and unavailable as well. As a result, a lot of my clients report being lonely as kids.

Many industries and marketing "gurus" I have been exposed to promote sacrificing now for a big future payoff, but that can come at the cost of relationships. Climbing to the top can be a lonely endeavor. And frequently, people get to the top and realize they are alone.

Traveling Job

Jobs that require a lot of traveling can be very hard on relationships, leaving people feeling alone and disconnected from their families, friends, and communities. It is hard to build quality relationships when you are gone much of the time.

Change of Job or Retirement

It is not unusual to see people in retirement return to the work world—finding they hated the unexpected boredom, lack of fulfillment, and loneliness they experienced in retirement. Financial instability may also lead a person to come out of retirement. I saw this happen with a lot of my fellow police officers who retired just in time to see the stock market crash and their 401(k)s plummet in the historic "dot-com bubble" burst that occurred from 2000 to 2001. They and many others woefully watched their investments and retirement accounts tank overnight, forcing them into new "retirement jobs." We saw it happen again for many who had invested in the housing market with the real estate crash of 2008.

Retirement or a change in jobs can affect relationships as well, especially when the change involves a move or a decrease in finances. Even in the best of circumstances, no matter what brought that change about, there is still almost always an adjustment in the depth of your relationships, at least temporarily, as you start over in your new environment. It takes time to let those friendships develop and deepen, and during that time, it is easy to feel lonely, missing the depth of relationships you once had in your old work environment.

Living Remotely

A person can choose to live in a remote area, making day-to-day interactions with other human beings more challenging and less frequent. Margaret lives an hour from the nearest city and 20 minutes from the nearest neighbor. Her husband farms, and her kids are grown. Though she loves living in a rural area, the development of close friendships takes ongoing face-to-face contact, and that has been difficult for her over the years.

Working Remotely

More and more people are working remotely, and while the convenience is nice, working from home has definitely increased feelings of isolation and loneliness in our society. Work relationships help us feel connected. If you are sick or have to miss work, co-workers are usually aware. It feels good to be seen—to have someone know the happenings in your life. These conversations happen in the workroom, in the staff lounge, by the watercooler, in restrooms, and in a shared office or pod.

As mentioned, close ongoing relationships that meet the needs of the heart require face-to-face interaction. Those office interactions can fill the extrovert's need for social interaction, and it is common for co-workers to become outside-of-the-office friends. Virtual friendships can happen through remote work, but they will not fully fill the heart's need for social interaction like physically being in the same office can.

Lack of Income

Whether by choice or circumstance, a lack of income can contribute to isolation and loneliness, especially if you are in an affluent community where many social activities come with a significant cost. Lack of income can mean less ability to participate in social connections that build community. I saw this play out in the schools, too, when I was a School Resource Officer. A student whose family income is low is limited in what extracurricular activities they can participate in.

Season of Life Requirements

Different seasons of life can play a part in contributing to feelings of loneliness. Debbie, a young mom with young children at home, struggles with loneliness because she feels trapped and overwhelmed by the day-to-day requirements of her young family. Not only is it a major ordeal to take her little crew out on an excursion, but the family has only one car, which her husband needs to get to and from work, so coordinating is challenging. If she wants the car, she has to get all of the kids up early, dressed, and into the car to take Dad to work. Then she has to repeat the process, interrupting naps, to pick him up. Because this is all so difficult, she rarely opts to have the car. She feels isolated because of the lack of adult contact, so she is very lonely.

Polly hates her career choice and is no doubt experiencing burnout. In an effort to be intentional about her situation and move herself into a more life-giving occupation, she has decided to go back to graduate school. So now, in addition to a demanding career, she has evening classes and homework. Not only is her situation unique from those around her, but her schedule is also tight and demanding, further worsening her feeling of isolation and lack of friends to connect with—even just to commiserate, debrief, and encourage one another.

And again, sometimes the challenge in a relationship is due to the lifestyle choices of another person.

For example, having friends or family move away can also cause loneliness. It is pretty common for me to see both friends and clients struggling with the issue of living away from family. Being an "empty nester" can be a painful experience for many parents.

Friendships take time to develop, and to have a portion of your life invested in a close relationship that ends up becoming a long-distance relationship can be very difficult. Not only is there a loss experienced in the day-to-day, face-to-face relationship, but there is also a very real loss in the support that comes from having friends and family living nearby. This can be devastating and cause deep feelings of loneliness. When this taps into earlier unhealed wounds of abandonment, it is all the more painful.

A WORD OF ENCOURAGEMENT

I've tried to make the point that loneliness is sometimes the result of choices we have made, but not always. I hope you can also see that loneliness is often about the situation a person finds themself in and not due to a flaw in the person. The good news is that in each decision, there is a strong possibility that you still have choices to be proactive and shorten the resulting season of loneliness. In taking responsibility, you can decide if you want to make changes or if you prefer to accept your circumstances and their consequences.

That said, extraordinary circumstances are sometimes a part of life—those things we didn't choose. Sometimes we play a part in them, but other times, life just serves up a tragedy that we did nothing to cause. Let's talk about some of those events in the next chapter.

CHAPTER 3

LONELINESS RELATED TO EXTRAORDINARY CIRCUMSTANCES

Sometimes, unexpected events leave us struggling with loneliness. They come with no warning. Adding to the trauma of these types of events, there is frequently nothing short of a miracle that can be done to change the situation. This can easily cause a person to feel victimized and discouraged, even struggling to feel much hope for a better life.

Additionally, it is not uncommon for a person to have a crisis of faith in such times. Deeply spiritual questions such as, "Where are You, God?," "Why did You let this happen?," "Are You even real?," and "Do You care about me?" often surface, adding misery to the struggle.

It doesn't help that some people seem to live charmed lives without much tragedy. Though you would never wish a tragedy on anyone, it can seem unfair that some people seem to lead almost magical lives while others have more than their fair share of crisis and tragedy. Though my life has been full of great richness and blessing, I am way too familiar with the extraordinary circumstances I have listed in this chapter and the struggle they bring. Maybe you can relate.

Perhaps you are struggling right now through an unavoidable circumstance. The loneliness can be overwhelming and add to your already trying circumstances. My heart goes out to you. I hope that as you read this chapter, you will feel seen.

Even though what you are going through can feel weighty and all-consuming, be encouraged. There are still things you can do to alleviate the enormous loneliness that can accompany such events. We will talk about those ideas in the next section, but first, let's identify what some of those extraordinary circumstances might be.

Caregiving

A person can feel quite isolated while serving as a full-time caregiver for a friend or family member. Additionally, the job of caring for a loved one sometimes requires relocating to an area where the caregiver doesn't know anyone, and the level of caregiving required can make it very difficult to leave the house and make new connections. (I share an encounter I had with the Lord about caregiving in Final Thoughts from My Heart at the end of this book.)

Illness or Lack of Mobility

Sometimes, your own extended illness can lead to isolation. In small towns or smaller churches, times of illness might be met with an outpouring of love and connection as friends come around to help. But often today, with the busyness of schedules, especially in bigger towns and megachurches, an illness can strand someone at home while no one really notices. A lack of mobility that makes it hard to get out and participate in social activities can do the same. Both can be isolating and lead to great loneliness.

Dietary and Other Accommodations

It can be hard to socialize with others when a person needs special dietary or environmental accommodations. That can be as simple (though not easy) as needing to avoid eating dairy or gluten, or it can be as challenging as having severe allergies or environmental sensitivities. These types of needs create challenges that can cause loneliness.

Mental Illness

Depression, Tourette's syndrome, social anxiety, agoraphobia, and OCD are just a few of the mental health issues that can challenge a person's social interactions and add to loneliness. Additionally, isolation can contribute to mental health issues. If you are friends with someone struggling with mental health issues, it can affect your own sense of loneliness when they self-isolate or randomly act out in ways that sabotage the relationship.

Physical and Mental Disabilities

Having a disability can isolate a person—especially if the person is dependent on someone else to transport them to doctor appointments, the grocery store, and other errands. The bus driver of an assistance van may be their strongest social connection. Sometimes, a disability can keep someone from getting out and about entirely. Social connections are limited to the phone or the internet, unless they are fortunate enough to have family nearby or friends who look in on them.

If you are disabled, lack funds, and have no family around, life can be very lonely. Even the most resourceful people may find many compounding factors too much to overcome, resulting in extreme loneliness.

Abuse

Abusive marriages and homes are often kept secret. That alone is isolating. But sadly, many abusive spouses also restrict their spouse's relationships with friends and family in an effort to control them. This restriction often applies to the children as well. Outside influences can serve to bring awareness that what they are living with is not normal or acceptable. Cutting off those outside relationships cuts off support, as well as any means of escape. This leaves a spouse and children isolated and alone to endure whatever is happening in the home. Whenever access to social interaction is cut off, the pain of loneliness, in addition to the abuse, is inevitable.

Death of a Loved One

The death of a loved one takes your heart into spaces of emptiness that are hard to describe. The loneliness created in the gap where once there was a treasured relationship is deepened by the great sadness that accompanies that loss. That sadness can be compounded by the way in which the person died. Both suicide and murder add huge complications to the grieving process, but any unexpected death can be devastating.

My daughter, Piper, died after an extended illness when she was fifteen years old. She was diagnosed with liver disease when she was three months old and was very ill until she had a liver transplant when she was five years old. Her life was fairly normal after her transplant but still involved daily immunosuppressant medication, regular visits to the doctor, continual medical tests, and lots of precautions.

We were well known at the local hospital, as Piper was there so frequently that she became a bit of a local celebrity. She became mysteriously ill again when she was thirteen. When she turned fifteen, it was discovered she was suffering from a rare form of organ transplant rejection—ten years after her original transplant. She was in the hospital for eight weeks before she died, so I had plenty of warning that the time was coming, but after she was gone, my brain still had such a hard time coping with how to plan moment-by-moment, day-to-day activities without making accommodations for her needs. It felt like there was a huge vacancy in both my head and my heart. I assume that is part of the shock you hear about that comes after a death. I was a single mom at the time and also had two wonderful boys, and I remarried two years later. Though my sons and husband Tom are just as special to me, no one could take Piper's place. Sometimes this mama's heart just misses her—and in that place, there is an emptiness that only she could fill.

Most people think losing a child is the hardest death one can experience, but I've observed that the loss of a spouse can turn one's life upside down like no other loss. Many widows and widowers struggle with loneliness in the aftermath of losing their spouse. If their spouse died of an extended terminal illness, oftentimes the loneliness comes a long time before the spouse dies. No matter how many friends you have, the death of a spouse ushers in tremendous loneliness.

Divorce and Breakups

Divorce can bring a lot of the same changes as the death of a spouse, but the ambiguity can be more confusing because the loss is of a spouse who is still alive. Whereas a widow or widower might feel abandoned by a spouse who has died, divorce often brings the pain of both abandonment and rejection.

To add to the confusion, many friendships are experienced as a couple. When there is a breakup or divorce, those relationships inevitably change. Friends may find themselves in the awkward position of having to choose sides or even withdraw from both individuals in an effort to avoid conflict. If kids are involved, it can affect their friendships, too. When a couple's relationship ends, everyone affected faces some measure of loss. That loss can potentially lead to loneliness—whether one was directly or indirectly affected by the breakup.

Traumatic Events and Disasters

It is not uncommon for a person to isolate themselves after experiencing a great loss or traumatic event. Just as a wounded animal will find a place to hide and be safe, people will often do the same. Sometimes, there is not enough emotional capacity after such a life-changing event to interact with others.

Surviving a disaster, trafficking, or being a refugee of war or violence often causes people to have to relocate—sometimes even to another country where they don't know the language. The level of trauma experienced can be inexpressible—especially to someone who has no way to relate to that person's experience. Rebuilding one's life after such extraordinary trauma can be overwhelming, and a person will often distance themselves to cope. This distancing exacerbates the trauma by adding a feeling of loneliness.

The Pandemic Effect

In the introduction, I talked about how research done during and after the COVID-19 pandemic lockdown showed a high correlation between an extended period of isolation and loneliness. The pandemic changed us forever. People shifted their work habits, their travel habits, their socializing habits, and even their churchgoing habits. The pandemic caused a lot of individuals to reorganize their lives, and not all of the shifts have been positive. Social scientists are now referring to the "friendship recession" in our country: People have fewer friends today than people had even a decade ago. In a day and age when communication and transportation have never been easier, the challenge of making new friends has become much harder.

Do you see a pattern evolving here?

When people feel they have experienced an out-of-the-ordinary event, it is easy to believe no one around them can understand what they have been through. In response, they may tend to withdraw into themselves, often unnoticed by the people around them. Feeling that no one truly knows and understands your world can be incredibly lonely.

A WORD OF ENCOURAGEMENT

Whatever the reason, the experience of loneliness is real. There are many factors that contribute to both physical isolation and the internal experience of feeling lonely. Most reasons have nothing to do with you as a person and have everything to do with circumstances. Understanding the reasons that contribute to loneliness can bring understanding and help you come up with solutions for either shortening the season or making the best of it.

Life can be hard, but that doesn't mean we are powerless. I once heard the actor Michael Caine share in an interview that if he had only one philosophy in life, it would be "Use the difficulty." Every person we admire who is wise and seasoned with maturity has walked through difficulty. This truth is even borne out in Scripture:

> Even in times of trouble we have a joyful confidence, knowing that our pressures will develop in us patient endurance. And patient endurance will refine our character, and proven character leads us back to hope. And this hope is not a disappointing fantasy, because we can now experience the endless love of God cascading into our hearts through the Holy Spirit who lives in us! (Romans 5:3–5, TPT)

You may just be trying to keep your head above water right now. That's okay. But hopefully by incorporating some of the ideas in this book, you will create a season in which you come out on the other side thriving. In Section 2, we will look at practical strategies you can implement to overcome loneliness.

SECTION 2

SOLUTIONS

WHAT YOU CAN DO TO BE PROACTIVE

SECTION 2 INTRODUCTION

WHAT TO DO IN THE MEANTIME

So how do you survive this season of loneliness—or better yet, how can you thrive? I believe you can.

I want to lay the groundwork for the ideas that follow with four different therapeutic techniques, skills that will help position your mind for love and growth:

- Listen to how you talk to yourself.
- Take a stance of compassionate curiosity.
- Acknowledge your feelings.
- Give yourself grace and acceptance.

Incorporating these four skills into every activity you engage in will bring you into a greater awareness of yourself, others, your circumstances, and the opportunities found in each. I highly recommend making these a regular practice in every season of your life—especially in challenging seasons.

1–Listen to How You Talk to Yourself

One of my favorite therapeutic techniques (and one I use myself) is to have my clients talk to themselves whenever they are discouraged, just like they would talk to their best friend. You can do this silently in your mind, or speak out loud, or write in a journal. Usually, that "friend's" voice sounds quite different and more supportive than the self-berating voice you have been hearing in your own head. I haven't yet had a client who, when asked to do this, didn't hear a different, more loving voice. An entirely different vocabulary comes out. The self-berating voice is exposed, and typically they realize how ugly and defeating it was. It begs the question, "Why would you talk to yourself in such a nasty manner when you would say entirely different things to a friend in the same situation?" All of us respond better to encouragement than discouragement. It's a great life skill to adopt—especially in a season of loneliness, when you may not have others to speak to and when the negative self-talk can be intense.

2–Take a Stance of Compassionate Curiosity

Another great technique utilized by both therapists and coaches is what is called "a stance of curiosity." Again, it requires ditching the negative internal voice, but this time trading it out for a position of curiosity in which you are simply observing your response in any given circumstance. I heard Dr. Gabor Maté call it "compassionate curiosity," and I loved that upgrade. It's about choosing to learn about yourself without judgment. It is amazing what we can see once we drop the self-condemnation and observe ourselves with grace. Replacing self-condemnation with compassionate curiosity when you are feeling lonely can open up awareness, which makes it easier to implement change—and it feels a whole lot better, too!

3–Acknowledge Your Feelings

Most of us tend to think our feelings are right or wrong. Have you ever found yourself saying, "I know I shouldn't be feeling this way, but …"? For some reason, we tend to have that perspective, and we "should" on ourselves—even if we have been taught feelings are neither good nor bad; it is what we *do* with our feelings that is good or bad. There is truth in that. Your feelings are just a necessary, God-given internal feedback system that tells you something is good or something is wrong. You may not understand why something bothers you so much, but it is in discovering the why that you gain an understanding of what you like and what you need.

Most of us have learned to discount our feelings—to push them down. Recognizing what you are feeling underneath that loneliness and giving yourself permission to feel those feelings goes a long way in healing the heart in a difficult season. Both *The Compassion Method* and *The Connection Codes* are two wonderful resources I use with my clients to develop this skill. (These are discussed in more detail in other places in this book and are also included in the Resources section at the end.)

4—Give Yourself Grace and Acceptance

Did you know that people tend to be far more successful at changing their behavior when they can love and accept themselves as they currently are? It is from that place of love and acceptance that they find the motivation to love themselves *better* through changing. It seems counterintuitive, doesn't it? Most of us think hating how or where we currently find ourselves is the best motivation to change, but how many times have you experienced failure to change when disgust was your motivation? Take losing weight, for example: In my health coach training, we were taught that it is hard to help someone lose weight until they come to love and accept themselves at their current weight. It is out of that place of acceptance that an energy is released, which provides the *sustained* goal of attaining a healthier weight. We see that play out in a lot of life arenas, not just with weight.

> NOTE: Are you a perfectionist? I used to be. It is an impossible standard that leaves you continually feeling like you come up short. It makes it really tough to give yourself grace and acceptance when all you can see are your failings.
>
> You have permission to give yourself grace because God does. God knows everything you and I will ever do. He understands us better than we understand ourselves, and He covered us with His Son (see John 3:16, Romans 3:23-24). The journey to knowing God as the God of this lavish grace is a life-changing journey that I encourage you to take if you struggle with self-acceptance. An impactful book that met

> me right where I was and helped me move from religious self-condemnation to grace was Andrew Farley's *The Naked Gospel*. I highly recommend it.
>
> Perfectionism is a problem that has both emotional and spiritual components. If you struggle with it, don't hesitate to get help.

So, what do these four tools have to do with loneliness? As discussed in Section 1, life circumstances can throw you into a season of being alone. What can you do? I hope to provide some ideas in this section, and these four techniques lay a foundation for each of the ideas I will share. When implementing any of the ideas in this book, look at how you are talking to yourself, take a stance of compassionate curiosity, allow yourself to feel your feelings, and give yourself a lot of grace in the journey—love and accept yourself right where you are. Loving yourself doesn't mean you will stop growing as a person. Quite the opposite! Self-acceptance lays the foundation and frees up the energy for positive change. Practicing these skills will help catapult you out of struggling and move you from surviving to thriving.

Let's start by looking at how to be your own best friend with ideas you can try on your own. In other words, learn how to be alone without being lonely!

CHAPTER 4

BECOMING YOUR OWN BEST FRIEND

Things You Can Do on Your Own

Doing things alone will never fill your heart in quite the same way that sharing activities with friends can, but that doesn't mean you have to be miserable when alone. Feel your feelings; it is okay to grieve. Just don't get lost in that place. Don't get stuck. There are ways to pull yourself out of that pit. Many who have come through loneliness will tell you that this time of being alone, or even just *feeling* alone, can still be a meaningful time. A season of alone time can have many benefits if you are open-minded and willing to use it to better yourself as a human being. You can explore ways to be comfortable with yourself and even entertain yourself when you are all you've got. It is in this process that you can learn to become your own best friend. This is a great life skill that will serve you well in the long run.

It is well accepted that learning how to be a good friend to yourself is the precursor to being a good friend to others. The Golden Rule even speaks to this: "Love your neighbor as yourself" (Romans 13:9). Make an effort to be entertained by this journey of life and where you have landed, making lemonade out of lemons for the pure moments of joy it can bring. Don't let this be a time of languishing! Challenge yourself with some of the suggestions in this chapter and see if you don't feel a sense of accomplishment after a while.

Use this time to become the person you want to be. What have you wanted to work on that you just haven't had the time or energy to do? The challenge of being overwhelmed and too busy will undoubtedly come back around. Take this alone time to water the seeds of your soul and experience growth that no one can take from you. I promise it will be worth it.

When this period of loneliness passes and your life fills with people again, you may even find you miss the solitude you made peace with (and maybe, just maybe, even came to enjoy). At that point, you may feel a desire to schedule more alone time back into your life. That may be hard to imagine right now, but I promise it happens!

OKAY, LET'S GET PRACTICAL!

Practice Gratitude

I start with gratitude because it is easy to do and takes only a small amount of effort to bring great gains. Gratitude is one of those "small hinges that opens a big door." You don't have to look very far to hear people sharing how adopting an attitude of gratitude changed their whole perspective on life. Several adults I know talk about growing up in a family that practiced going around the table at dinnertime and each sharing a gratitude for the day, and it is a treasured memory for them now. Others I know have adopted a daily habit of listing things they are thankful for in the morning and again at the end of the day, both opening and closing the day with positivity and joy.

Well-known author Francis Frangipane is often quoted for what he has written about gratitude:

> *The very quality of your life, whether you love it or hate it, is based upon how thankful you are toward God. It is one's attitude that determines whether life unfolds into a place of blessedness or wretchedness. Indeed, looking at the same rose bush, some people complain that the roses have thorns while others rejoice that some thorns come with roses. It all depends on your perspective.*
>
> *This is the only life you will have before you enter eternity. If you want to find joy, you must first find thankfulness.*

Indeed, the one who is thankful for even a little enjoys much. But the unappreciative soul is always miserable, always complaining. He lives outside the shelter of the Most High God.

[...] Most of us simply need to repent of ingratitude, for it is ingratitude itself that is keeping wounds alive! We simply need to forgive the wrongs of the past and become thankful for what we have in the present. The moment we become grateful, we actually begin to ascend spiritually into the presence of God.

> NOTE: It is true, gratitude ushers in the presence of God. Psalms 100:4 says, "Enter into His gates with thanksgiving, and into His courts with praise. Be thankful to Him, and bless His name" (NKJV).
>
> Using the tabernacle as a metaphor for His presence, the psalmist writes that thanksgiving gets us into God's presence. Praise takes us deeper still into intimacy with Him. Thanksgiving is gratitude for what He has done. Praise is the expression of gratitude for who He is.
>
> I start every session with gratitude, asking my client to share something they are grateful for, and then I offer that gratitude to Him with praise. God taught me to do this. There is a promise of His presence in this practice! It makes such a difference.

When a person feels lonely, their thoughts tend to focus on what they don't have. Gratitude helps lift our thoughts up and keeps us from drowning in despair. Thinking about what you are grateful for provides balance to those thoughts of what you lack, sometimes even replacing them. It is simple but powerful. Additionally, when you feel all alone, gratitude has a way of pulling in thoughts of people who have contributed to your life. And though they may not be currently in your life, you are surrounded by blessings that others had a part in, and that can help stir up the belief that others do care about you.

Practice Being in the Present with Mindfulness

When loneliness threatens to overwhelm you, it can be helpful to practice mindfulness. The internet is full of mindfulness activities to try. One of the most effective mindfulness tools I've used with clients struggling with anxiety is called the "5-4-3-2-1 Tool" developed by Betty Alice Erickson. You move into an awareness of the present and mentally observe five things you can see, four things you can feel, three things you can hear, two things you can smell, and one thing you can taste. Those can be currently present or recently experienced. It is a great exercise for bringing your thoughts into a very present state. I suggest it for any time you are struggling with the negative, repeating thoughts that can often accompany loneliness. (It is also a great tool if you find yourself dissociating as either a coping response to discomfort or out of habit.)

God impressed upon me once that regret and worry serve the same purpose—they both take us out of facing today. Being present is important, but sometimes your present circumstance when you are feeling lonely can feel insurmountable or overwhelming, and so the tendency can be to resort to the distraction of either regret (over things we have experienced) or worry (over future things we imagine). Recognizing that neither regret nor worry offers any valuable contribution to your life and typically just fills your head with negative thoughts can be a good motivator for practicing mindfulness and getting comfortable with the uncomfortable in the present. Staying present in your loneliness is certainly not an easy path, but it is a courageous one. And it is the path that will lead you to the answers you seek. Regret and worry will not.

Reset Your Vagus Nerve

Are you familiar with the vagus nerve? It is the longest cranial nerve in the body. It plays a part in regulating our heart rate, breathing, and digestion. The vagus nerve gets dysregulated by long-term stress, trauma, lack of sleep, inflammation, imbalanced gut health, and chronic illness—issues that often accompany loneliness. Resetting the vagus nerve can rebalance your entire nervous system in a way that allows your body to physically help combat the low mood that comes with loneliness by lifting your mood, increasing a sense of peace, and elevating your overall sense of well-being.

There are simple ways to help reset the vagus nerve. My personal favorite is humming. Other techniques that can be effective include deep breathing, meditation, cold exposure (cold plunge, cold shower, etc.), singing, laughing, or a throat and neck massage. The results can be powerful. I have more ideas available at https://leslieparkertaylor.com (see Resources).

Take a Break

I can't overemphasize the value of taking breaks. I have learned personally how valuable they are. They add joy to life, prevent and remediate burnout, and keep a person healthy.

No doubt, life is busy, and finding time to carve out a break takes intention and conviction. Give yourself grace. Quiet the head noise and realize you cannot be all things to all people. Without proper refueling, your effectiveness in everything you are passionate about will be affected. If you struggle to find some time to refresh and renew, apply some compassionate curiosity and figure out whether you are dealing with legitimate reasons or just excuses.

> NOTE: There is some great research done by Dr. Sahar Yousef, a cognitive neuroscientist, which she has called the "3M Framework." She found that taking what she called *maxo breaks* (a half day to one full day a month), *meso breaks* (one to four hours per week), and *micro breaks* (a few minutes several times a day) can revitalize a person struggling with burnout. I have found this powerfully true in my own life and very highly recommend this practice to many of my clients. Here are some examples of each:

> ***Maxo Breaks***: every month, a half day to one full day
> Examples: Leave your environment for a day in nature, take a hike or a day trip to somewhere beautiful, have a picnic with a good book, or spend time with a friend.
>
> ***Meso Breaks***: every week, one to four hours
> Examples: Getting out of your regular routine can help you to recharge. Enjoy a hobby; participate in a sport; garden; cook a special meal; go for a bike ride, a walk, or a short hike; visit a park, museum, library, or bookstore; or meet a friend for coffee or lunch.
>
> ***Micro Breaks***: every day, a few minutes several times a day
> Examples: Make time to pause and refresh. Close your eyes for a few minutes, give yourself a head massage, focus on deep breathing, take a quick walk, take a short power nap, stretch or do a quick round of high-intensity interval training, practice a mindfulness exercise (e.g., 5-4-3-2-1), make a cup of tea, meditate, worship, or sit with the Lord.
>
> Dr. Yousef emphasizes that taking a break does not mean scrolling on your phone or checking email. It should be a true psychological break, the equivalent of time at the beach.

A period of loneliness can be emotionally difficult. Finding some intentional ways to engage in enjoyable activities—even if those activities are done alone—can be additional "small hinges that open big doors" for bringing joy back into your life. And if you can find joy during a time of aloneness, imagine how much greater the joy will be when your situation shifts. You will be a joy expert!

> NOTE: Blake K. Healy, currently Director of Bethel Atlanta School of Supernatural Ministry, has had the ability to see both angels and demons since he was a young child. In his third book, *Indestructible* (mentioned in Chapter 1), he speaks from the perspective of a seer about the value of fun and rest in becoming "indestructible" to the Enemy. (I went to ministry school with Blake and highly recommend his books.)

Laugh

We've all heard it said that "laughter is the best medicine." That applies to the heart as well as the body. The power of laughter has been respected by medical and spiritual experts for centuries. As early as 900 BC, King Solomon, a king known for his wisdom, wrote: "A joyful, cheerful heart brings healing to both body and soul. But the one whose heart is crushed struggles with sickness and depression" (Proverbs 17:22, TPT).

Beyond the benefits of joy, a good, full-hearted laugh relieves stress and muscle tension and boosts immunity. It stimulates many of your internal organs and is especially beneficial to the lungs and heart. Laughing releases endorphins and increases oxygen intake, both of which activate the parasympathetic nervous system, reducing stress. Muscles stay relaxed for up to forty-five minutes after a good laughing session.

Norman Cousins was a well-respected author and university professor who taught ethics and medicine. He was particularly interested in the effect of emotions on health, and he even used humor to beat the 500:1 odds of being cured of his connective tissue disease and ankylosing spondylitis. Cousins discovered that if he belly laughed for ten minutes, he could sleep pain-free for at least two hours. When the effect wore off, he would watch a comedy film, laugh some more, and buy himself another two hours of sleep without pain. He penned a number of books on the topic of health, but his most famous is *Anatomy of an Illness: As Perceived by the Patient*, in which he shared the experience of his illness.

Many doctors prescribe laughter for their patients. It literally changes the chemistry of the body. In a season of loneliness, your body chemistry isn't at its best. While battling all the "sad chemicals" that can come from being unhappy, see if you can integrate laughter into your life and give your body that boost of positive chemicals to counter the sad ones. This can go a long way in helping you feel better and thrive.

Challenge Your Negative Thoughts

Negative thoughts naturally accompany loneliness—but they don't have to. (I will talk about negative thoughts several times in this book because mindset is so important.)

It helps to realize that negative thoughts are a natural product of our "primitive brain" (the brain stem and limbic system, including the amygdala, hippocampus, hypothalamus, and thalamus), which is geared to protect us at all costs. The first step is to become aware of negative thoughts. The wonderful

Dr. Daniel Amen calls these "automatic negative thoughts" or ANTS.

So how do you combat those ANTS and turn them into what he calls PETS (positive empowering thoughts)? Awareness is the first step. Next, you trade them out for prearranged positive statements or declarations (or a Bible verse). Here are some examples:

ANTS	PETS
"I'm not good at this."	"Every master was once a disaster!"
"I'm so stupid."	"Everyone makes mistakes. I don't have to be perfect."
"I can't do this."	"I can do all things through Christ who strengthens me."
"This is hard."	"This is new."

That last one comes from my own life. A business coach once said to me, "Leslie, why do you keep saying, 'It is hard'? Why not just say, 'It is new?'" That was a light bulb moment for me, a complete reframe for whenever I run into something I want to label "hard." More often than not, it is just new! I was expecting mastery before it was time.

There are circumstances that come into play in a season of loneliness (discussed in Section 1), and then there are your thoughts about those circumstances. If all of those thoughts were positive, one could argue, "Would you feel lonely?" How we view our circumstances is always more of a determinant of our experience than the circumstances themselves. History, as well as the many personal stories we hear of people overcoming incredibly difficult circumstances, shows this to be true.

Changing a negative mindset to a more positive one takes awareness, intention, and time. Have grace for yourself. Talk kindly to yourself. Be compassionately curious, noticing what seems to tip you more into a negative mindset. Being tired or hungry (ever hear the term "hangry"?), experiencing a conflict or disappointment of some sort, not feeling well—all can contribute to negative thinking. Notice when you are most vulnerable. See if there is a pattern to it. Then you can be ready to grab those thoughts and take them captive or reframe them. (See more on negative thoughts in Chapters 5 and 6.)

Get Outdoors

Sometimes you just need to get away from all of the carpet, laminates, and linoleum in your home and office and get out into the greenery and fresh air of nature. There is something wonderfully refreshing and renewing about getting out in nature. There are beautiful waterfalls within an hour's drive from where I live in northern California. Hiking and mountain biking trails are plentiful. Just a short walk from my home, there is a trail that goes along the Sacramento River for over fourteen miles. Places like these in nature never get old and always seem to refresh the soul.

There are documented health benefits tied to getting outside into nature as well. These include improved mood, a sense of calm and relaxation, better sleep, boosted immunity, increased cognitive function, and a reduction in mental fatigue and stress. Exposure to sunlight has also been shown to increase levels of vitamin D, which is deficient in most Americans. A deficiency in vitamin D is associated with depression and anxiety. Wouldn't it be interesting to find that your struggle with sadness in a season of loneliness is more a matter of vitamin D deficiency than circumstance?

Have you heard of "earthing" or grounding? Earthing is connecting your bare feet directly with the earth's surface—grass, dirt, sand—such as in a park or on a beach. Preliminary research findings offer promising support for the possible benefits of earthing, benefits long held as truth by natural health practitioners. It is believed that this practice facilitates the exchanging of electrons between the body and earth, which results in a reduction of free radicals and inflammation in the body. Benefits include improved sleep, pain reduction, stress reduction, and an overall improvement in well-being—all of which can build resiliency in a season of loneliness. When we feel better physically, we feel better emotionally. We also feel more hopeful, which increases our desire and capacity to be proactive.

It takes discipline to stop what you are doing and go outside, but getting outdoors (barring inclement weather or bad air quality) is a practice with immediate benefits.

Get Moving

They say "sitting" is the newest health crisis. Researchers are talking about how valuable not just exercising but simply moving itself can be to our sedentary device-focused, television-watching lifestyles.

Studies have shown there can be tremendous health benefits from walking just ten minutes three times a day. In addition to the physical health benefits derived from movement, research shows that walking twenty minutes a day is also associated with lower levels of loneliness and social isolation.

Ideas for movement that do not require another person include gardening, yardwork, housework, gym workouts, stretching, hiking, walking, running, and bicycle riding. Whether you're going to a gym, doing virtual workouts, or exercising on your own, it is important to add movement to your routine to thrive in a season of loneliness.

Practice Self-Care

While all of these ideas lend themselves to good self-care, I want to mention self-care as a separate point of focus to emphasize its importance. So often our lives are lived according to what we think everyone else needs from us. And in a season of loneliness, it is easy to get swallowed up in self-pity. This is a good time to listen to your own needs. Maybe it's your physical health that needs attention. Maybe it's your mental health. Perhaps it is your connection to God.

Have a good check-in with yourself, practicing a little compassionate curiosity. What are you needing? What has been neglected? What needs attention? Be your own best friend. Give yourself grace, accept where you currently are, and then start caring for yourself! I promise you'll reap big benefits!

Whether or not you are married, have lots of friends, or are raising a family, you are responsible for taking care of you.

Have you ever gone without seeing someone for a long time, and then when you finally do see them again, they look amazing? When we take good care of ourselves, we feel better (and the compliments are nice too). Good self-care shows. Whether you are hoping to make new friends or simply want to feel your best, good self-care will set the foundation for everything else. Remember, like attracts like. Who do you want to attract? Be a good friend to yourself, and you'll attract people who value you at the same level you value and care for yourself.

Get Healthy

Having a season that is not saturated with social engagements and their accompanying diet-violating temptations can be a good time to focus on another way to love yourself better—using it as a time to get healthier. I'm a big fan of what I call the "Big Six." Scientists tell us that more than 80 percent of all health issues could be eliminated if we just focused on improving these six areas: sleep, water intake, movement, good nutrition (including supplementation), detoxing (eliminating toxins), and mitigating stress.

So many issues connected to loneliness are outside our control, but optimizing our health is not. When we are healthier, we are happier—whether we're lonely or not.

> NOTE: My husband and I used to believe that if we ate a variety of healthy, organic food, our nutritional needs would be met. However, we have since learned from some scientists we came to know that our food is not as nutrient-rich as it once was. (Research that, it is shocking!) In today's world, we need to fill in this nutrient gap with high-quality, bioavailable supplements. We followed their advice and were shocked to experience the difference! (For more information, see my website listed in the Resources section at the end of this book.)

Work on Personal Growth and Self-Reflection

There is a wealth of personal growth and self-education resources available online and in most communities. Watch for local events sponsored by libraries, churches, community groups, colleges, and universities. Platforms like Kindle Unlimited allow you to cycle through a variety of books and magazines for a low monthly fee. Many local libraries also offer an online service that allows you to check out ebooks for free. A couple of apps I am aware of in our area are Libby by Overdrive and Hoopla. A self-paced personal growth journey might involve a journaling habit, self-help books, personal growth groups, podcasts, videos, workshops, online training, classes, and/or the help of a coach, mentor, or therapist.

> NOTE: I would be remiss if I didn't add that there is no better way to work on personal growth than pursuing God. He is the best personal growth coach you could ever have! You want to become a better version of yourself? Pursue a relationship with Him. He promises that if you seek Him with all of your heart, you will find Him (Jeremiah 29:13). Ideas for pursuing Him include talking to Him, reading about Him, spending time in His Word (the Bible), worshipping Him, contemplating Him, and *pressing in* to know Him more.

Investing in your personal growth can make the emptiness of a lonely season less empty. A good metaphor is a cocoon birthing a butterfly. Hard seasons usually make us better people. Invest this time in the journey for yourself and see who you become on the "other side." Did you know that if you get 1 percent better every day, you'll be thirty-seven times better in a year? That's an increase of 3,700 percent! Baby steps, baby; they count!

Connect to Your Heart

I have had the chance to both witness and experience how healing it is to give attention and permission to what your heart is feeling.

Most of us are taught to disregard our hearts from a very early age. Have you ever been told one of these phrases: "Buck up," "Put on your big girl panties," "Stop crying," "Don't be a cry baby," or "Quit whining"? We may even be encouraged to disregard our hearts with optimism, with statements such as "It will all work out," or "You'll be okay." Sometimes it even has a good Christian spin on it: "God will make a way," "Nothing is impossible for God," or "God will bring it to good." Do any of those sound familiar? We hear it from our parents, teachers, preachers, and friends. Pretty soon, we are saying it to ourselves without even realizing we are shutting down the voice in our own hearts. In the process, we use our heads to process our pain rather than our hearts. The result is a heart that is shut down and a brain that is stuck ruminating on our experiences.

When your emotions are triggered, your heart is trying to tell you something. The best practice is to go to your heart and ask it what it is feeling. This can take practice, so give yourself grace as you develop the skill. I've found the voice of my heart speaks in simple terms with no accompanying explanation. It just shares what it feels. It will say something like "I'm tired," "I'm overwhelmed," "I'm angry," "I'm afraid," or "I'm embarrassed." As the heart shares what it is feeling, you can dig deeper by asking it, "And what else?" This is a good habit, as the heart usually has more to say when given the attention. I liken it to "draining the pond"—getting all of the reactive emotions out.

Laura Duncan's *Compassion Method* teaches that under all the reactive emotions, there is always one of three "tender emotions": sadness, fear, or loneliness. The three are like conjoined triplets and are often hard to pull apart, but after identifying all the reactive emotions, if you ask your heart which one of those three tender emotions it is feeling the most and just sit with it a moment, it will usually tell you.

Once you have identified the tender emotion underneath, you can speak to your heart and give it permission to feel what it is feeling using language like "I understand why you feel that way," "It is okay to feel that way," or "You can feel that way as long as you need to." That last phrase was a hard one for me to embrace. I was afraid I would get stuck in that feeling, but I found that is not what happens.

Acknowledging what your heart is feeling and then giving it permission to feel that emotion opens a door to healing. I'm convinced it opens a major pathway for the Holy Spirit to come in and do His healing work. Sometimes you can even feel it happen, but most of the time, it is more of a progression of healing.

> NOTE: There is a great deal more to Laura Duncan's *Compassion Method*. It has a second component that is excellent for healing earlier wounds that are still affecting us. If connecting to your heart in this season appeals to you, find a certified *Compassion Method* consultant, like myself, to work with. Laura's website has a link to her podcast and workbook, as well as a list of her advanced certified consultants (see Resources).

Pursue Creativity

Research shows that when you are super lonely, something in your brain opens up to allow for greater creativity. What a great time to write that book or screenplay! Use the time to learn a new craft or even shake the dust off a craft you used to enjoy but haven't done in a while. Ideas abound on social media and the internet. Nothing like creating something that will take your thoughts to a more beautiful place. If you can have fun with it, give yourself grace and put aside those perfectionist tendencies. Creating can also be a great stress reliever by reducing cortisol levels, so it's good for your body and brain. The sense of accomplishment can also be deeply satisfying. You could even share your creations with others and earn some income through your own website or Etsy.

Creativity can find expression in every area of life. It is limitless! Some traditional ideas include cake decorating, candy making, baking, needlework (crocheting, needlepoint, embroidery, knitting, etc.), woodworking, pottery, ceramics, photography, quilting, rug making, canning, and painting. Less common ideas include calligraphy, paper crafting (like origami), paper cutting or quilling, jewelry making, and basket weaving.

Inspiration can be found on social media, Facebook (Meta), Instagram, and Pinterest. You can find so many ideas there for yard and home decor, activities for kids, and bringing new life to old furniture and other discards.

Local businesses, community colleges, and libraries offer classes. These can be a great way to meet new people. Usually the groups are small, so it isn't as overwhelming for an introvert or shy person. (More on this in Chapter 5.)

Start a Collection

Starting a collection can open up a whole new fascination and give you the opportunity to add pleasure and mental stimulation to your life. For some collectors, there is the bonus of creating a legacy, which can give purpose to one's life.

I collected coins as a child, but as an adult, I enjoy collecting beach glass and heart rocks. My husband would tell you I actually collect rocks in general—I find it hard to resist small rocks that catch my eye, and occasionally, an extra special larger one makes it home.

Collections can also create social opportunities. They often make for interesting conversation and connect you with people of like interest. They can even set the foundation of a meaningful friendship. Collections can also provide special gifts between collectors. For someone who loves what you do, a gift from your personal collection can be a special treat.

> NOTE: A word of caution: We know that collecting can help satisfy that emptiness that comes with loneliness, making it a great activity in this season, but beware. There is some evidence that when some people feel extremely lonely, that satisfaction can become an obsession, ending up both isolating and bankrupting them. Don't let that be you. Enjoy collecting, let it open whatever exciting doors it might, but also be aware and keep a watchful eye.

Engage in Hobbies

Hobbies can provide some of the same benefits of creativity and collecting. They can also bless others. My friends' hobbies have blessed me in so many ways—my cousin Teresa's scrapbooking, her husband Dan's drawings as they travel the globe, my friend Becki's paintings always shown "in progress," and my friend Mel's incredible wildlife photography—all of them regularly post their work on social media. They all live a long distance from me, but they still bring such delight to my day when their hobbies pop up in my feed.

Several clients have shared with me incredibly meaningful songs and poems they have written. They are so deeply moving and really impact me. It is okay to have a hobby just for personal enjoyment. Even better, consider if you have a hobby that might bless someone else. Admittedly, sometimes it takes a little bravery to share, but there can be great pleasure in bringing that joy to others, and that sharing can open up exchanges that bring social connection in a lonely season.

There are many hobbies you can pursue. Maybe this list will inspire your own ideas: cooking/baking, antique shopping, thrift shop adventures, reading, gardening, painting, drawing, composing music, doing puzzles, writing (poems, screenplays, books, articles, ads, blogs, etc.), scrapbooking, stained glass making, woodworking, candle making, furniture refurbishing, and metal detecting (this one has always intrigued me).

Give Attention to Your Home and Yard

What have you not had time to do around your home—organizing your home, making or arranging for repairs, deep cleaning, painting? If you are renting, you will have more limitations on what you can do, but are there things you need the landlord or management company to be aware of? It can be hard to find the time to do these kinds of maintenance jobs. Partnering with someone you know who has the skills you need can make it easier, plus it can build a fun connection. Sometimes a professional can do a much better job.

It can be a challenge to find the time to make the phone calls to hire someone to do home repairs. Use this as a season of catching up. It feels so good to have your home in order. It makes it easier to feel comfortable inviting others over as well. How many people decide to fix up their home just before putting it on the market only to wonder afterward why they didn't fix it up for themselves? Be your own best friend and do it for yourself now! Anything and everything that can bring a spark of joy will help brighten a season of loneliness.

If actually doing the work is not an option right now, here is another idea: clip photos of home or yard ideas you like. I'm very drawn to videos and photos of home and yard projects. In fact, the photo albums on my phone and my Pinterest account are full of saved ideas. I ponder on the various ideas for years with a lot of joy until I feel the go-ahead to implement them.

Get That "Other" To-Do List Done

There may be no better feeling than one of accomplishment. If you find yourself in that awkward "in between friends" season, it can be a great time to create and check off a few items on that to-do list. Your list might include ideas to improve your life, such as setting a budget or retirement planning. Maybe it is time to create a vision board and start going after those things you want for your life.

For those of us who are a little older, the list might also include those end-of-life to-dos no one likes to think about but that will be such a big help to those you leave behind. These might include getting your estate in order (with a will, power of attorney, end-of-life instructions, etc.), organizing your affairs, and cleaning out your home—culling through all of the excess you may have accumulated yourself rather than leaving all of that for your heirs to manage.

How about creating a legacy to-do list? What do you want to show for your life after you are gone? Maybe your family is your legacy, and you have been busy building that. But maybe you have dreams of creating something tangible that will bless others when you no longer can. This season can be a good time to ponder on those thoughts, dream a little bit more, and put those ideas in action. If this appeals to you but you don't know where to start, don't be afraid to hire a life coach.

> NOTE: It is easy to feel disappointed if you do a life review and realize what you thought you would have accomplished by now hasn't happened. To that, I want to say this: *You are enough!* Goals and dreams can be wonderful, and they have their place, but even if you never do anything but show up each day as a kind and loving person to those around you, you are making a valuable contribution to the world, and your life matters. Living in the present and being your authentic self leaves an incredible legacy in the hearts of every person you encounter.

Learn a New Musical Instrument or Language

Learning either a new musical instrument or a language will add new neural pathways to your brain while also giving you the joy of accomplishment. Both can open up avenues of connection with others, too, as you find common ground in what you are learning. This can be a good time to take lessons, either one-on-one or in a group setting. With one-on-one training, there is the enjoyment of developing a strong relationship with your teacher—a person who sees you every week. With a group class, you have the benefit of meeting and interacting with other people who are trying to learn the same skill. Practicing a new language also opens up other opportunities to get together with classmates outside of class to practice. Of course, it can require a lot of grace for yourself. Mastering something new can take time. I love the saying "Every master was once a disaster!" It can be helpful to remember that.

To me, an instrument is almost like a pet. There can be a lot of solace there when you need to lose yourself for a little bit. Perhaps you have an instrument gathering dust in your house. This could be a good time to pull it out, brush off the dust, and make a little music—maybe even write a song!

Learn a New Tech-Related Skill

The world of technology is changing rapidly, and there are a variety of classes out there, both online and in person.

These might include learning how to use all of the features on your smartphone or taking better photographs with your phone. You can learn a new software program, such as Outlook or PowerPoint, or learn web design. The world of artificial intelligence (AI) has exploded recently, with plenty of opportunities for learning. Best of all, these skills are marketable. Not only are computer skills frequently listed as desirable on many job postings, they are also skills you can use to freelance for additional income on sites such as Fiverr.

Using this time to better yourself and your skills can bring not only entertainment but also fulfillment and purpose to life. This season won't last forever. Use this time to enhance what you know, who you are, and what you can contribute to the world.

Travel

Traveling alone can feel a little daunting, but listen to your inner talk. If you find yourself thinking, *That's too hard*, replacing that thought with, *It's just new*, can help. For those who are brave enough, travel is an excellent way to add adventure and new connections to a season of loneliness. Online travel communities can introduce you to other solo travelers. I have several friends who have "cruise buddies"—strangers who hit it off on a cruise and decide to do other cruises together. That said, the appeal of travel is not solely for the opportunity to make new friends but also to have fun on your own. You don't have to wait for someone to invite you or for another person to go with you.

A quick internet search of the phrase "solo travel" will turn up quite a few travel sites that organize fun tour groups strictly for solo travelers. The idea is to "travel solo but not alone." I recommend including in your search phrases relevant to you, like "solo woman travel," "solo senior travel," or "volunteer travel," to get you started on planning a solo travel adventure.

Adopt a Pet

Animals make great companions, and the research supporting the physical and mental health benefits of having a pet is prolific. Owning a pet can lower blood pressure, reduce stress, drop cortisol levels, help manage anxiety, depression, and PTSD, boost mood, and improve sleep. And you know what else it relieves? Loneliness! It is not surprising that eleven million Americans acquired a new pet during the pandemic. Maybe a pet dog or cat is not for you, but other popular pets include rabbits, ferrets, guinea pigs, rats, hamsters, lizards, iguanas, turtles, horses, chickens, ducks, miniature pigs, fish, snakes, gerbils, birds, and geckos.

—Take Your Dog to Obedience Class

If you already own a pet, this can be a good time to teach them some new tricks. If you own a dog, look for a dog obedience class in your area. These are usually fun to participate in as puppies and older dogs try to figure out what their owner wants them to do. Their different personalities come out, too, which is cute to watch. I've taken several dogs through dog obedience classes and have fond memories of the experience. I can still remember this one adorable old English bulldog in one of those classes who left a large puddle of drool every time the trainer had us give our dogs the command to sit.

—*Foster a Pet*

If you are leery of pet ownership, consider fostering a pet. Many local animal shelters have fostering programs so homeless animals can receive temporary love and attention while they are waiting to be adopted. It can give you not only companionship but also a sense of purpose and contribution.

I recently heard of an organization called PAWS (Pets Are Wonderful Supports). They have a program called PALS (Pets and Loving Seniors) in which people over sixty-five who have a limited budget and live independently can foster a dog or cat. PAWS retains ownership of the animal and pays for its food, supplies, and vet bills. A quick internet search pulled up many variations of this program in multiple cities. If you or someone you know fits the criteria, this can be an affordable way to have a pet companion when your/their budget otherwise wouldn't allow it.

—Train a Service Animal

Another possibility is to look into becoming a trainer for a service animal. You've most likely seen dogs wearing small red vests designating them as service dogs in training. Dogs can be trained for a number of services, including as guide dogs for the visually impaired or hearing dogs for the hearing impaired. Top breeds trained for service include golden retrievers, Labradors, German shepherds, collies, and poodles.

Dogs and cats can also serve as emotional support animals, providing support for individuals with various physical and mental conditions. Almost any dog breed can serve as an emotional companion dog and may be designated as such without special training. (Be aware that the laws for emotional support animals are different from those for service animals.)

If training a service animal interests you, it can open up an entirely new world of connections, both through the training community and pretty much anywhere you go with the dog. Training a service animal can not only give you a sense of purpose, but the animal also acts as a natural connector. Have you ever seen the videos of a guy sitting on a bench by himself while people are walking by? Then they give him a puppy and all sorts of people stop to chat with him and his dog. I have to say, this worked for my husband when we were both still single. He would come to our singles' events with his puppy, who was struggling with some health issues, and everyone was drawn to him and the puppy. I witnessed the magic of the dog connection with my own eyes!

> Fun Fact #1: The Americans with Disabilities Act (ADA) also recognizes trained miniature horses as service animals.
>
> Fun Fact #2: There is evidence that simply watching cat videos can elevate mood.

Make a New Friend—Connect with a Professional Listening Service

In the past, it was not uncommon to hear of friendships that were developed through pen pals—individuals writing letters back and forth. Did you know that you can connect with someone on a regular basis over the phone as well? There are several listening services out there. There is no location restriction, and some are even free of charge. If you are looking for meaningful conversation and this appeals to you, check the internet for what is available in the way of professional listening services and select the one that is the best fit for you.

> NOTE: As a therapist, I quickly came to realize that sometimes a person doesn't need therapy so much as they need a space to talk things over and be heard. To meet this need, I created A Listening Friend. It is staffed by some of the best listeners I know, personal friends of mine whom I hand-selected for this purpose. You can find more information on our company in the Resources section at the end of this book.

Seek Professional Support

If you feel like despair is growing and nothing you have tried is helping, or if you lack the motivation to even try any of the ideas in this book, it might be time to employ the services of a mental health professional. Professional counselors can now serve people both in person and online through video appointments. As a therapist, I was originally very skeptical about the effectiveness of virtual therapy, but after several years of doing video sessions, I've been overwhelmingly delighted with how well it works.

> NOTE: If you have an interest in working with our team, I currently see clients at the Transformation Center, a church-based counseling and inner healing center in Redding, California. We have an entire staff of pastoral counselors and clinical therapists who can see clients both in person and by video (see Resources for more information).
>
> I also occasionally work with a very small number of private consulting clients online. For more information on that service, you can connect with me by email or through my website at https://leslieparkertaylor.com (see Resources).

A WORD OF ENCOURAGEMENT

A season of being alone can be difficult, but on the other side, people can often look back and see a wealth of good that came from it. Keep your eyes wide open for the good things this season can bring, and realize you are powerful. Tony Robbins, a well-known motivational speaker, says, "Trade your expectations for appreciation, and your whole world changes in an instant."

We are created for connection, and the need to belong is a basic human need. Yet learning how to become your own best friend and developing the ability to be alone without getting lost in loneliness is a powerful life skill that will set you up well in life. More importantly, that sense of completeness is probably the single greatest factor in attracting others who are healthy and whole themselves. In the next chapter, we will talk about ideas for doing just that—building community!

CHAPTER 5

CONNECTING WITH OTHERS

How to Build Community

Years ago, I noticed there were two types of people in the church we were attending: those who thought the church was cold and unwelcoming and those who thought it was wonderful and were making a lot of friends. The difference? Those in the first group were waiting for someone to invite them over, to include them in activities. Those in the second group were proactive. They didn't wait for an invitation; they started inviting people to connect. The distinction was obvious.

I started seeing these same behavior patterns play out in other groups. Those who were proactive created community and readily felt like they belonged. Those who were waiting for an invitation were more commonly disappointed and expressed a negative perspective toward the group they were hoping to belong to. Their experience might be quite real. Certainly, some churches and groups of people are friendlier and more welcoming than others, but I think the principle holds true and is worth keeping in mind—if you want community, you have to be proactive in developing it.

I find this attitude can be reflected in how people view life in general. Some people let life happen to them and always live in response to their circumstances. Others believe they are powerful enough to design their own world and take action to create the life they want. For Christians, that action is partnered with God. That's not to say that events don't happen in our lives that we have no responsibility for, but there is so much that we can do to affect how our lives turn out. There is no better illustration of this than in the battle to overcome loneliness.

It is true: Simply putting the effort into building community doesn't mean it will be easy or even work in some scenarios. My clients have shared with me that sometimes they feel like they have put a lot of effort into developing friends and still cannot get people to respond. This is a valid experience, but the principle still applies. You have to take responsibility for your life if you want things to change, and this takes courage and resilience.

> NOTE: This, to me, is where personal faith can play a significant role. You are not alone in your efforts. God created you to be in a community. He wants this for you. It may take longer than you like. It may be harder than you want. He may feel more distant than you can bear. Maybe you even feel abandoned by Him. I know that is super painful. I want to encourage you to not give up. As you continue to press in, as you keep your face toward Him, you will find answers. Sometimes what He is doing on your behalf is in the unseen realm, and His timing can be different from ours. We know His ways are higher than our ways (Isaiah 55:9). Offer gratitude for any small shifts: insights you get, creative ideas that come, a small wind of refreshment, a glimmer of hope, a day that feels easier than the day before, an accomplishment you can see. He uses every piece of our lives (Romans 8:28). He is the God who gives beauty for ashes (Isaiah 61:3), and He will use this season to develop new strength in you.

Taking those realities into account and realizing there can be challenges, let's talk practically about what some proactive efforts can look like in building community. There are two directions you can go. One is reconnecting with people you already know, building on relationships that already exist; and the other is building new connections with people you don't know (yet!).

OKAY, LET'S GET PRACTICAL!

Let's first talk about ideas for reconnecting with people you already know. Sometimes, you can put in a good effort and still struggle with getting a response. My suggestion would be to give some of these ideas a try. Don't sabotage yourself with overly high expectations, which can lead to disappointment and frustration. Enjoy each interaction for the event that it is. Use your effort as a filter of sorts to see who wants to connect and simply needs someone to take the initiative. You can also feel good about being proactive. The advantage of starting with people you already know is the time that has already been invested in the relationship.

IDEAS FOR RECONNECTING WITH PEOPLE YOU KNOW:

Reconnect with People from Your Past on Social Media

At a time when a lot of my friends are dropping off social media, I still find it such a nice way to connect with what is happening in friends' lives—both local and at a distance. Before social media, I had completely lost touch with classmates I had grown up with and considered good friends. It was fun when I joined Facebook and reconnected with old friends some thirty years after losing contact. Both Facebook (now known as Meta) and Instagram have provided a good way to keep up with family too. It's nice to follow what everyone is doing, and commenting or sending private messages via social media is one way to stay connected. Reconnecting opens doors for video calls and travel, as well as for reigniting old friendships. It is not the same as being in the same town, but it can do a lot for the heart to reconnect with old friends who share some history with you.

Even for people living in the same town, social media can be just as effective. I have friends here in town whom I rarely see anymore because our lives have taken such different paths, but we stay connected on social media, oohing and ahhing over engagements and marriages, new babies and grandbabies, travels, and movies or events not to miss in the community. It's not unusual for friends to schedule a coffee or lunch date after connecting on social media.

Write Handwritten Letters and Cards

This is an art that has fallen by the wayside with the advent of texting and email, but letters and cards are still a delight to receive. Handwritten notes have a way of connecting hearts in a way that typewritten emails or texts just can't quite capture. It's not unusual for someone to save the cards and letters they receive from loved ones. That speaks to how much they are treasured. What a great legacy of love to leave behind too! Being alone offers time to do things like this that might be a greater challenge when your social calendar fills up. I certainly fall prey to the ease of sending a quick thank-you via text, and while that is better than nothing, a handwritten thank-you card always conveys a deeper level of appreciation.

You can sit down and spend a day sending out cards and letters, or you can set a goal that feels meaningful and attainable, like sending out a letter or card to one person every week. Choose the option that best reflects your passion for the idea, and make or buy stationery that reflects your personality and style.

You never know what might come of it. Another friend of mine started writing to an inmate to encourage him. What started out as correspondence between pen pals turned into a friendship that eventually led to marriage—first behind bars and now for many years happily at home together.

Reinvest in Groups You Are Already In

Almost every group has volunteer opportunities. Where are you around people who already know who you are? Is there an opportunity there to jump in and serve? Serving with others is a fun way to make deeper connections with people without the strain of coming up with things to talk about. The "job" you are volunteering for often comes with conversation. Volunteer for jobs that involve others rather than one-person projects. Be honest with the coordinator and let them know you want to use the opportunity to get to know people better.

Most churches have Bible classes and smaller group opportunities. In a smaller church, you may already know people and see a lot of familiar faces. In a larger church, it may be an opportunity to meet new people. Some of the opportunities you might see in churches include:

- women's or men's groups
- mothers of littles and mothers of middles groups
- Bible studies
- Sunday morning and midweek Bible classes
- home groups
- communion preparation
- volunteering in ministry or prayer groups
- answering phones
- helping in the office or kitchen
- ushering, decorating, setting up, or tearing down for regular and special events

Engage More Deeply with Co-Workers

Work and school environments frequently have a variety of ongoing projects that need volunteers (e.g., office parties, community projects, fundraisers, etc.). These can provide a great opportunity to meet up with co-workers to discuss ideas or to work on the project together.

Lydia's daughter was a student in a private school. Lydia frequently saw the other moms as they came and went, dropping off and picking up their kids. When a big fundraising event was announced, Lydia signed up to help. Doing so helped her to get to know some of the other moms better—and she quickly discerned who she wanted to spend more time with.

If you feel nervous about inviting a co-worker out for coffee, remember that a majority of people are experiencing loneliness right now. Your co-worker may be just as delighted as you at the possibility of getting to know each other better!

It's interesting to get to talk to people behind closed doors like I do as a therapist. I know the majority of my clients struggle with loneliness, and they are amazing people who are invested in personal growth and want to be the best human beings they can be. As I mentioned before, they aren't lonely because of some personal character flaw. It is common for people to have the sense that everyone is getting together except them, but I think that perception is off. From where I sit, most people are struggling to make friends they can socialize with.

Sometimes, the best "cure" is to quit thinking about what might be wrong with you or why you weren't invited and start doing some inviting yourself. When you're at work or engaging in an activity at your church or in your neighborhood, pay attention to who is not in the group conversations. You have to look for them; they don't stand out. Invite them to lunch or coffee. All you have to do is say you'd like to get to know them better and leave it at that. Again, no heavy expectation for what it might lead to. Making new friends takes some effort and time. Start the filtering process with small invites to see whom you might click with and want to spend more time with.

IDEAS FOR MEETING ENTIRELY NEW PEOPLE:

Explore Online Communities that Share a Similar Interest

This can be done through social media groups and pages or through private groups started by people who share your interests. Sometimes you will see a small monthly fee attached to groups that are run by a coach or trainer, but often, especially on social media, you can access different communities entirely for free.

Many trainings and support groups are now offered online. While these connections are most likely to develop into online relationships and not local ones, you may be surprised how quickly you can make a connection with a stranger through the internet!

Mary and Sally both signed up for a four-week writing class organized by a mutual friend. They didn't know each other, but when the instructor sent the class into break-out groups of two, they partnered with each other. They found they instantly connected well, and they became fast friends. They live in different states, but since meeting in that online class, Mary has visited Sally at her home several times, and they even roomed together once at a Christian women's conference. (Mary confessed later that she usually clicks out of trainings any time they go into break-out groups, but this training was too small to get away with doing so. Obviously, she is very glad she stayed in!)

Some online communities you can join on social media include:

- book groups
- alcohol ink painting groups
- rock painters
- cyclers
- runners
- pickleball players
- rock collectors
- DIY groups
- seniors
- support groups for a wide variety of issues, from cancer to weight loss to narcissistic abuse

Each group offers a space to ask questions, share tips, give and receive encouragement, and show off something discovered, read, or created.

Local marketplace pages on social media can also be a fun place to connect sellers and buyers of household goods. Different pages can give recommendations for local establishments like restaurants and repair services, all of which open the door to new opportunities for local connection and relationships.

Join a Local Support Group

As mentioned, a lot of support groups now meet online, but local papers and community magazines will often list support groups that meet in-person in the community:

- AA (Alcoholics Anonymous)
- Al-Anon
- NA (Narcotics Anonymous)
- OA (Overeaters Anonymous)
- TOPS (Take Off Pounds Sensibly)
- MOPS (Mothers of Preschoolers)
- Divorce Recovery
- Grief support groups

Any of these can be a great place to meet people going through a similar experience as you.

Meet with Others Who Share Your Passion

You can find schedules for various local interest groups in community publications or posted online. In our community, there are all sorts of in-person groups focused on:

- books
- pottery
- ceramics
- alcohol ink painting
- rock painting
- quilting
- hiking
- pickleball
- cycling

If you are older, senior citizen centers often have activity calendars and are known for hosting bingo and ping-pong tournaments.

My friend Christine and her sister LaVerne joined a local "rockhounding" group. They go rock hunting in a new location every month with the group, bringing home treasures—rocks unique to that particular area. The leader of the group coordinates where they will go each time. Christine and LaVerne come home exhausted but with their hearts full, having found great rocks and also having met new people who share the same passion.

Take a Class in the Community

Most communities of substantial size offer a variety of classes throughout the week. If they are not listed on a community bulletin board, they can be a little challenging to find. Libraries, community colleges, and universities are a good place to start.

Some craft-related stores like Hobby Lobby or Michaels often offer classes. I took a beginner's cake decorating class at Michaels years ago. It was fun. After the Carr Fire in California destroyed my friend Mary Joy's home, I took her to an alcohol ink painting class. (Alcohol ink is a type of ink, not to be confused with an alcoholic beverage.) We had a memorable time, and it turned out to be a refreshing break from all the somber realities of the fire.

These types of activities tend to be very social. You can certainly go into them quietly, keeping to yourself, and go home without meeting anyone (I've been known to do that), but if you are motivated to make new friends, they usually create a fun atmosphere that is conducive to getting acquainted (and laughing a lot!).

Join an Exercise Group

The local YMCA can be a good place to go for group exercise classes. A friend I know teaches a water aerobics class there. Our community senior center hosts ongoing ping-pong games, and many gyms will host classes (which may carry a cost on top of the cost of gym membership). Examples of group exercise opportunities include the following:

- running clubs
- cycling groups
- Barre classes
- step classes
- spinning
- aerobics
- swim aerobics
- hiking groups

Some communities offer small exercise studios. We have a fitness center here that is part of a larger franchise designed exclusively for women called Curves. It creates community for the women who go there throughout the week. CrossFit is very popular here, too, and I know a lot of people get pretty tight with their CrossFit "family."

Dana, an exercise instructor at a gym, found a local group in her community that gets together once a month to do some outdoor activities. Sometimes they ride their bikes together. Other times they go on a hike. It helps get her outside and moving. It has also brought new friends into her life.

Pickleball is a big craze in our community (and many others). While retired persons may have more availability, I hear of more and more young people enjoying the sport. David is someone who packs his pickleball paddle every time he travels. He shows up at the local courts and always finds people willing to work him into a game (it is accepted pickleball culture to do so). His love of pickleball is not only giving him exercise, but it is also making him new friends everywhere he goes.

Become a Community Volunteer

Every community has volunteer opportunities. Find an activity you are passionate about, and make sure it involves working with other people. Here are some ideas of places to volunteer:

- the local animal shelter
- the library
- CASA (Court Appointed Special Advocates for children)
- foster care

- trail cleanup
- graffiti cleanup
- beach cleanup
- city council
- the school board
- the school's PTA (Parent Teacher Association), if you have school-aged children

My client Denise is a Court Appointed Special Advocate (CASA) for kids. It doesn't pay anything, and most of her relationships there do not spill over into her personal life, but she would tell you it is the most fulfilling thing she does. It gives her life meaning and satisfaction when so many other aspects of her life seem to be in flux. She loves her volunteer job so much, she structures the rest of her schedule around it.

Elevate Your Social Skills

Practice building your confidence at social events. If you, like me, are a little introverted at events, it can help to have a good mindset. Keep your focus on other people. We have a tendency to focus on our own discomfort, and that only makes things worse. Go with someone, if you can. Having someone to show up with can help with that initial awkwardness most people feel when they go to an event full of people they don't know well.

Look for people who are standing alone and who may need someone to talk to. Use the FORM technique, asking them about their <u>F</u>amily/<u>F</u>riends, their <u>O</u>ccupation, their <u>R</u>ecreation/interests, and (if you get that far) their <u>M</u>otivation. (You can find more information on the FORM technique on the internet.) Match their body language. Ask open-ended questions. Be upbeat and positive. Humor is usually a nice icebreaker; it feels good to get someone to laugh. And most importantly, show genuine interest.

> NOTE: Need some help with this? Check out *I Hear You* by Michael S. Sorensen. It is a great book on validating people and can go a long way in easing social anxiety and helping you develop meaningful relationships.

Start a Home Group

You don't typically need permission to start a group in your own home. What sounds fun to you? A Bible study group? A dinner group? Maybe just a group that meets for fun?

Our good friends Dave and Maryann have a high-quality big-screen television. They are much better at hosting social gatherings than my husband and I are. Every year on Super Bowl Sunday, they host a Super Bowl party. Dave smokes a brisket, and everyone else brings a side dish or two. It's a lot of fun. We didn't know the other people who were invited at first, but now we do. By opening their home, Dave and Maryann expanded everyone's friendship circles. What a gift!

Whenever you host an event, it has the potential to include and bless others.

My clients Carl and Chloe started a Bible study group in their home. It became so popular that it eventually grew into a church!

Carmen and Ray started a dinner group with three other couples they wanted to get to know better. Years later, the four couples remain close and still meet for dinner once a month.

Bobby and Margaret host regular movie nights where they take turns choosing a movie. Everyone gets advance notice to approve or disapprove of the choice.

Charlotte and James host game nights where they play various card games. Similarly, you might prefer to host small gatherings to play board games.

Billie wanted to invite connection into her life but didn't have room for gatherings in her small condo. She sent out a letter to her neighbors asking who was interested in playing bunko, and now they meet weekly at their condo clubhouse to play, with everyone pitching in on the small rental fee.

Be Proactive

Let me end with the same message I started with—be proactive.

My friend Harrison and his wife, Linda, recently moved to our city and have already built a community of good friends. Harrison has a strict boundary about going to bed at 8:30 p.m. because he knows he'll feel better in the morning. That seriously limits their options for attending evening social events. To their credit, Harrison and Linda are very hospitable with their home and frequently host group activities—but everyone knows they have to leave by 8:00 p.m. No one minds (though some have to be encouraged toward the door). Because Harrison and Linda are proactive in meeting their social needs in a way that works for them, they don't wrestle with issues of loneliness.

That invitation you keep waiting for (that might never come)? Try being the one who gives it. The best part about doing the inviting is that you already know you'll be part of the group!

Look for people who might also be in a lonely season. Look for people you have things in common with or just enjoy being around. Invite them for a coffee, lunch, or a walk, with no expectation to turn it into anything more. Do it just to meet more people, to get out of the house and spend time with others. If you are ministry-minded, do it to serve others. Who knows what might come of it?

I've had clients complain that they have invited a new acquaintance to coffee and then couldn't get them to do much beyond that. I know doing the inviting doesn't always solve the challenge, but it at least puts you in control and increases your chances of building relationships.

A WORD OF ENCOURAGEMENT

It's a little cliché, but it's true—the only way you can fail is to quit. It may take more effort than you wish it would. You may get discouraged. But do not give up. You simply cannot fail if you keep yourself encouraged and don't stop making an effort toward connection.

Perhaps the greatest challenge in reaching out is the fear of rejection or failure—two of the biggest fears people have. If you find that either of these fears is holding you back, give yourself grace, acknowledge the fear, and recognize that you can't engage more socially without some risk. Find the ideas in this book that feel the most doable, and remember that baby steps count. And don't forget to celebrate the small victories; they will be worth it!

In the next section, we'll turn the focus more toward the individual—things to consider and watch out for, as well as areas you might want to shore up within yourself as you use this season of loneliness to become your best self.

SECTION 3

CONSIDERATIONS

HOW TO OPTIMIZE AND NOT SABOTAGE YOURSELF

SECTION 3 INTRODUCTION

A FEW THINGS TO CONSIDER

A lonely season is never easy. In Chapter 6, I want to shine a light on the self-destructive choices we commonly see people gravitate toward in an effort to find relief from the distress they are feeling. My hope is that with a heads-up, you can prevent going in that direction.

In Chapter 7, I discuss ways that you might be contributing to your current situation. I was hesitant to include this chapter because there are so many complicated outside factors that contribute to loneliness, and people tend to blame themselves enough as it is. But it seemed like a good opportunity to do a self-checkup, taking an honest look at any behaviors you might be able to improve on. If the goal is to make friends, then while we are looking at ways to connect with other people, why not also work on becoming a better friend? In this chapter, I point out problematic behaviors, but if you find yourself in one or more of them, don't worry; I also offer suggestions. I hope this chapter both challenges and blesses you.

Lastly, in Chapter 8, I share my thoughts on when you should consider seeking professional help. I have included this because I get asked this question a lot when I train disaster workers. As a therapist, a certified health coach, a pastor, and a life-long learner committed to my own personal growth, I am aware of a variety of healing modalities that tap into different areas of our well-being—mental, emotional, physical, and spiritual. I don't think you need to be hurting to benefit from healing work in these areas. This chapter is included as a nudge, though, to seek help if you are struggling. You are not alone.

CHAPTER 6

SELF-SABOTAGING COPING BEHAVIORS

We are told there are two main motivators in human behavior: pain and pleasure. We tend to move away from pain and toward pleasure. As human beings, we tend to want to self-medicate to escape pain. In our minds, it may satisfy both needs—bring pleasure and stop the pain. If we can reduce the pain, why not? The problem is that the short-term solution is often not the best long-term solution, and sometimes what we turn to for relief of pain in the present only causes more pain in the long run.

When Redding, the California community in which I live, experienced the devastation of the Carr Fire—over 1,000 homes burned to the ground in July of 2018—disaster workers from the Tubbs Fire in Napa Valley (which had occurred the year before) came to help and share what they had learned from their fire. At the time, their fire was the most destructive wildfire in California history, with 5,636 structures destroyed and 22 lives lost (later surpassed by the Camp Fire our team deployed to in Paradise, California, in November 2018, which destroyed 18,804 structures—11,000 of which were homes—and killed 85 people).

One thing the disaster workers from the Tubbs Fire shared with us was the surprising number of disaster workers who turned to drugs and alcohol to cope with the stress. This information gave us the opportunity to be proactive with our disaster workers; we encouraged them to find positive activities to relieve the stress of the disaster instead of falling into the temptation to self-medicate with drugs or alcohol. The same applies to any challenging season. Avoid the pitfalls that can cause greater problems down the road.

There are many ways we can self-medicate. I've included in this chapter a list of the most common self-sabotaging coping behaviors I've seen people use to escape their pain. My purpose here is not to get caught up in the moral argument surrounding these but to give you a heads-up on signs to watch for. Let your own moral compass be the guide, and set up accountability with someone if you need it.

I think it is also important to note that every one of the "cautions" given in this chapter is related to what we are thinking about. Our thoughts are the precursors to our behaviors. It is vital to pay attention to our thoughts. When we change our thoughts, we change the neural pathways in our brain. Dr. Caroline Leaf and Dr. Daniel Amen are two of my favorite authors who write on the importance of our thoughts, how to take control of them, and how they interplay with the neuroplasticity of our brains. (Check out the many books they each have written if you want to learn more on this topic. Their websites are listed in the Resources section.)

As discussed in previous chapters, there are so many healthy options to explore in a lonely season—options that bring opportunity for both connection and a better life. Don't let the pain you are experiencing right now lead to behaviors that bring immediate relief but accentuate your discouragement and delay true relief.

OKAY, LET'S GET PRACTICAL!

Substance Abuse

We are a society that likes to avoid pain at all costs. Self-medicating with alcohol, cigarettes, and drugs can be very costly, however. They are an easy go-to when stressed, usually bringing some level of immediate relief, but they often open the door to a boatload of more pain. No one expects to get addicted, but it happens. All of us have seen it. And loneliness opens a wide door to addiction. An addiction to drugs, cigarettes, or alcohol has never served to better anyone's life;

it only serves to create more loneliness and alienation. The best option is to stay away from things that lend themselves to chemical addiction. If you find yourself already struggling with substance abuse, don't be afraid to enlist help and take action.

While earning my master's degree, I attended a number of Alcoholics Anonymous (AA) groups. One of the groups I attended was full of businessmen and women who worked downtown. All of them had been sober for many years, and I learned a lot from them. While I believe that with God it is possible to get entirely free of an addiction, one of the tricks they used to get free and stay free of their craving for alcohol was to substitute that addiction for a healthier one. Many of them became runners; if they felt like drinking, they put on their running shoes and ran until the urge passed.

Physical exercise is usually an effective alternative, but it's not for everyone. A friend of mine who quit smoking found she initially needed to keep her hands busy, so she took up crocheting. She successfully kicked the habit, and a lot of family members got personally crocheted gifts from her that Christmas!

I believe the principle of substitution is a valid one for some people on the road to recovery. A new, healthier obsession can offer you a stepping stone out of a more damaging addiction and be easier to break than a habit of drug or alcohol abuse.

If you find it hard to stop on your own, I recommend getting help through a recovery group like Alcoholics Anonymous (AA) or Narcotics Anonymous (NA) or connecting with a personal Certified Addictions Counselor (CAC), aka a Certified Alcohol and Drug Counselor (CADC) or Alcohol Drug Counselor (ADC), depending on where you live. If you are struggling, don't believe the lie that you can do it on your own. There are so many people who have been where you are, and they are dedicated to helping others get free. I'll say it again: you are not alone!

Excessive Shopping

There is something a little bit intoxicating, even exhilarating, about buying new things. It's fun. But if the purchases exceed your budget, it can bring a whole lot of woeful stress down the road when that credit card bill is due and your utilities still need to be paid.

Bonnie found that spending money on others and eating out with friends soothed the loneliness she felt in her marriage. That comfort was short-lived when she had to pick up extra hours at work to pay off her credit card bill. The accrued debt didn't help her marriage, either. The extra work, decreased social time with her friends, and increased tension in her marriage all made her loneliness worse.

Some ideas to curb excessive shopping include going window shopping and leaving your phone and credit cards at home.

Go with a friend for accountability, or shop at a dollar store (where at least the shopping will do minimal damage). Take turns with friends hosting lunch rather than going out—or go out for coffee instead of a meal. Many of my friends also like to walk and talk—which is free!

Pornography

Pornography addiction is an epidemic—even in the church. It doesn't help that the resources are as close as your phone or computer. There is plenty that could be said about the travesty of sex trafficking in our world and how this is so tied to pornography. For our purposes, it is important to recognize that at a time when you are trying to build connection, this is the ultimate activity that reinforces seclusion. From my experience as a therapist, I can tell you that it is addicting, and it destroys relationships.

If you're struggling with pornography addiction, consider putting controls on all your devices. Commit to honesty with those closest to you, and have someone to hold you accountable. Set boundaries that create success. Get therapeutic help for what is driving the root cause—and get educated about sex trafficking.

> NOTE: Aaron Zint produces good resources that deal with overcoming a pornography addiction. He has a podcast and a book, both titled *Numb to Known*. He also runs small online recovery groups. I went to ministry school with Aaron and his wife, Jenna. They are doing a lot of fun things to help people improve their lives (see Resources).

Poor Self-Care

Who in a time of busyness or stress can't relate to having let go of established healthy routines at some point in time? Poor self-care can show itself in a variety of ways—any way that neglects the body, soul, or spirit. Letting yourself go never makes anyone feel better, and getting back into good habits of self-care admittedly can be a chore.

Do what you can to keep those good habits going in this season. In fact, as discussed further in Chapter 7, this can be a great time to *increase* your self-care. Pouring into your own well-being is rarely wasted time and can go a long way in keeping your spirits up during a lonely season.

> NOTE: *Atomic Habits* by James Clear is one of the best books for implementing new habits you want and extinguishing old ones that don't serve you. Jenna Zint also has a very popular Habit Lab (see Resources).

Isolation

For those who are introverted, this is a tough habit to break, and it has gotten only tougher since the pandemic. It can be hard to get out and do things with other people, especially if you don't know them well. The easier thing to do is isolate, but then the misery that accompanies loneliness only grows. Relationship expert Love McPherson says our "social muscle" atrophied during the pandemic. It is important that we rebuild that muscle. It's okay to pace yourself. Give yourself grace. Baby steps count. Just keep in mind that stretching yourself to interact with others will pay a big reward.

Me-Focus

It is so easy to fall into the self-pity pit. All our focus can be on ourselves, how victimized we feel, and how disappointed we are with where things stand in our current circumstance. God told me once that He is not always on the throne of my life. I was horrified and would have argued, except He planted a knowing of the truth in my heart at the same time. I was focused on something; I can't remember what it was, but it was consuming my thoughts. God told me that thing was on the throne. Then He paused and told me that sometimes I am on the throne. The realization was honestly so repulsive to me, and I realized in that moment how much of my thoughts were on myself—even in ways I thought were good, like pondering, *Was I as considerate as I should have been? Did I dominate the conversation? Was there more I could have done? I need to start exercising! I wonder why I wasn't included? No one sees my potential. I feel pigeonholed. I'm so tired*, and *I'm so discouraged*. All those thoughts were focused on *me*!

It can be like turning a train around to get your thoughts off yourself, but when I notice what I am focusing my thoughts on and realize that thing is currently sitting on the throne of my life, it convicts me. When those thoughts are persistent, I declare that God is on the throne of my life, and I go to Him for help with those thoughts. Sometimes it is a battle, but it's one worth fighting.

It can be so natural to focus on ourselves. It is the exceptional person that truly doesn't. Even the person who is always giving to others may be coming from a codependent place, where the root motivation underneath is really about the self (i.e., to be liked, to be well thought of, to feel good about oneself, etc.). I want to encourage you to observe your thoughts and not lose this season by having a me-focus and missing out on all the things He wants to do in you. This can deepen the pit and make crawling out all the harder.

The Blame Game

It is easy to get stuck on blaming others in life when things are not going as we would like—especially in a season of loneliness. Blame is often justified, but it is also a distraction. It puts our focus on others and often leaves us feeling powerless in our circumstances. There is room for accountability, brave communication, and the setting of boundaries. But getting stuck in offense and blaming others for our situation doesn't solve anything. It certainly doesn't move us out of loneliness. Realizing the role others play can be important to sort out, but then it is important to move into productive problem-solving. Do you need to forgive? Let go of offense? What can you change, and what must you accept? The more options you see for yourself, the more empowered you will be. And the more empowered you are, the more you will thrive in *any* season.

Here is a great quote by Henry Wadsworth Longfellow I really love that can help with blaming: "If we could read the secret history of our enemies, we should find in each man's life sorrow and suffering enough to disarm all hostility." Such a powerful thought!

There is always a reason people behave as they do. It doesn't mean it is excusable. Boundaries and consequences may need to be put in place, but the internal choice to hold on to blame only hurts us further.

Negative Thoughts

Though I talked about negative thoughts in Chapter 5 and will do so again in Chapter 7, I mention it here as something to watch for. When we are lonely and discouraged, it is easy to fall into a pattern of negative thinking.

In college, I learned about the concept of "metacognition." I found it fascinating. Metacognition is the awareness of your own thought processes—or thinking about what you are thinking about. It can be helpful in a difficult season to put checks in place to notice what you are thinking about. Journaling can help with that. Simply taking time to stop and be aware can be useful. Remember, as you listen to how you talk to yourself, do so from a stance of compassionate curiosity, acknowledging your feelings and giving yourself plenty of grace and acceptance (see Section 2). What you focus on is what will grow!

> NOTE: With those thoughts in mind, pick a topic, a person, an event, or an object that continually has your attention. Get out a notebook or journal and draw a line down the center of the page. On the left side of the page, write your free-flowing thoughts about it. Are they full of negativity or positivity? Do you want to be a more positive person? Start writing all the positive attributes on the right side, then train your thoughts to stay focused on that side (see Philippians 4:8).

Losing Hope

Almost every client I have who struggles with loneliness also struggles with hoping their situation will change. Author Francis Frangipane says, "Any system of thinking that does not have hope, which feels hopeless, is a stronghold which must be pulled down." Several of the pastors in my church teach that any area of our lives not glistening with hope is under the influence of a lie that steals one's vision of a good future.

Hopelessness is a lie. Break agreement with it. Speak the opposite of what you are feeling over your life. Partnering with hopeless thoughts only increases loneliness. Remember, with effort, loneliness is a season that will pass. You are powerful, and you can effect change.

Depression

Focusing on what isn't happening, whatever is a disappointment in your life, can be a slippery slope into depression. If you start to realize depression might be creeping into your life, it's best to get ahead of it as soon as possible.

Several non-pharmaceutical solutions have been found to be quite effective for preventing and treating depression. For example, research has shown that one of the best ways to beat depression is by serving—getting out and volunteering for a cause that benefits others.

Equally effective is spending some time finding what brings you pleasure, what gives you a sense of accomplishment, and doing more of that.

Exercise can help depression as well. Dr. Josh Axe shares that walking forty-five minutes a day, four times a week, is as effective as antidepressant medication after twelve weeks and *more* effective after ten months (see Resources).

Depression can take you down a deep, dark pit. If you feel loneliness is leading you into depression, stop to consider your thoughts. If you struggle with turning them around, get professional help (see Chapter 8).

A WORD OF ENCOURAGEMENT

It is easy to get discouraged in a hard season. It is especially easy to get discouraged when you are feeling alone. Listen to how you talk to yourself. Love yourself well. Take care of yourself. Watch out for the pitfalls and put the brakes on them early. Most importantly, give yourself grace and hold on to hope.

> NOTE: For Christians, our hope is found in God. Romans 15:13 (NLT) says, "I pray that God, the source of hope, will fill you completely with joy and peace because you trust in Him. Then you will overflow with confident hope through the power of the Holy Spirit." Hope requires trust, and I know that for many, trust is a challenge because God doesn't promise to protect us from hard experiences—quite the opposite. James tells us that we should be thankful for trials, that they build endurance (see James 1:2-3). They are not especially fun, but we can trust God. The point is to not give up hope and to not give up doing good. Galatians 6:9 says that we will reap a harvest from the seeds we plant. Hope comes from believing that.
>
> I realize that throwing Bible verses at our struggles can only add to the pain for some people. On the other hand, if we hold the Word of God as truth, then we can lean into it even when we do not have full understanding of it. Proverbs 3:5-6 (NLT) says, "Trust in the LORD with all your heart; do not depend on your own understanding. Seek His will in all you do, and He will show you which path to take." Whenever I get discouraged, even when I get stuck there for a time, this is a verse that helps pull me out. Like a ladder against the wall of a deep, hand-dug well, He is always there to help us crawl out of the pit, rung by rung—if we are willing to partner with Him.

Do you still think you might be a defective human being? I would argue that you are a perfect representation of the human species, with a lot to offer. We are all in process and will always have room to grow, especially as it relates to our relationships with others. With that in mind, the next chapter will provide you with an opportunity to look inward (not with shame and condemnation but with compassionate curiosity and grace) and identify common behaviors that could be hindering your best efforts to connect with others.

CHAPTER 7

TAKING PERSONAL INVENTORY

As I mentioned before, every client I have who struggles with loneliness wonders if there is something wrong with them. Loneliness can cause you to feel like a social outcast. It can be a feeling of being on the outside looking in—looking into a world where you see others socializing but feel yourself outside of those activities, unable to get in.

Rarely to never is the issue something my client is doing wrong. They are not the social misfit they may perceive themselves to be. Sometimes they know they are not, yet deep down inside there is that quiet little voice that questions why they feel so lonely, wondering why people don't seem to want to be with them.

I'd be remiss to write this book and not look at some of the ways our own behaviors can contribute to our feelings of loneliness. Certainly, as we saw in Section 1, if you identified with any of the reasons listed, you know that some things in our circumstances cannot be helped—but some can! This chapter is included to help you look at common personal social habits that may be contributing to your experience of loneliness. Remember, as you read through this chapter, if you identify with some of the behaviors listed, love and accept yourself in your current circumstance first. Give yourself grace. There is always an understandable reason for why we are the way we are.

I must admit, I'm familiar with a lot of the behaviors listed here because I've been guilty of many of them. They can be hard habits to break. I've found that what starts hard suddenly gets easier when I'm with someone who excessively displays that same behavior toward me (for example, interrupting). It's eye-opening! It's the perfect motivation I need to stop. I like to think I have recovered from most of these, but reminders are always good. If you find yourself relating to anything in this chapter, you're in good company.

OKAY, LET'S GET PRACTICAL!

Egocentrism

Egocentrism is the perspective that the world revolves around you. Most of us would never admit that this describes us, yet it's pretty common. When we move about in social circles with our people-pleasing ways and self-protection in place, our focus is actually on ourselves. Can you see that?

This comes out in conversation too. Do you ever catch yourself thinking about the next thing you are going to say rather than fully listening to what the other person is saying? Maybe you have been around people who always turn the conversation back to themselves—*their* thoughts and *their* experiences.

I've caught myself doing this when I feel a personal connection with what someone is sharing, and I think that by sharing my story, they will feel that connection as well. Sometimes that is true. It is an artful dance that requires a great deal of social intuition. More often, though, the other person feels sidelined when what they're talking about gets derailed before they are done saying all they want to say. I bet you've had that experience. You weren't really finished sharing about your own experience when the other person redirected the conversation to themselves. We may be eager to share about ourselves, but sometimes that can be a turnoff.

When you get into a conversation, dial down any thoughts about the impression you will make. Make a good impression by showing a genuine interest in others. Have a mindset to *understand* rather than respond. Be ready to learn all you can about the other person—what they are doing, what they are thinking, how they feel about things. There is truth to Maya Angelou's observation: "People will forget what you said, people will forget what you did, but people will never forget how you made them feel."

Talking a Lot

Let's face it. Some of us just talk more than others. Some of us have more thoughts swimming around in our heads, pressing to get out. But have you ever been in a small group, a class, or a team meeting where one or two people seemed clueless as to how much they dominate the discussion? I'm sure you have. Almost every small gathering of people has one. The drive to share may come from a need for attention. It may come from having an overabundance of ideas to share. It may even come from a discomfort with silence or an effort to give the leader some good responsiveness. Whatever the motivation, they often seem to be completely unaware that by dominating the time, they are taking away the opportunity for others to contribute to the discussion.

One of my biggest pet peeves is going to a lecture of some sort to hear an expert speak on a particular topic, only to have their time side-swiped by someone in the class raising their hand and then taking five to ten minutes to share something about what they know. I appreciate when a speaker can manage people in the audience who do this, but as a speaker myself, I know it can be a challenge.

It doesn't only happen in group settings; it happens in one-on-one conversations, too. And while there are a few quiet individuals who are truly grateful to have someone else doing all the talking, most people will leave such a conversation feeling uncared for, undervalued, and annoyed. I used to leave social situations berating myself for talking so much. I still need to watch for it. A good friendship is one in which the conversation is balanced. Though some occasions may call for the focus to be on one person, if it is frequently imbalanced, the relationship will often suffer.

> NOTE: When someone is isolated at home, caring for small children, or taking care of someone who is ill, you may find they talk a lot when they get out socially. To be seen and heard is a basic human need, and in their day-to-day life, they may be giving so much to others who need their attention that when they get out socially, they themselves appear needy. They are simply hungry to be heard by someone, anyone. Love these people if you have the capacity. These seasons are usually temporary. Hopefully with time, they will have an epiphany, like I did.

Oversharing

Have you ever sat next to someone you just met, and the next thing you know, you are privy to all their medical conditions and/or their family drama? That will run people off. People may be kind and polite and listen well, but they most likely won't invite that person over for coffee anytime soon.

Tom and I had this happen on a weekend trip to the coast recently. When we arrived, we were so excited to get out on the beach for a few minutes and just enjoy a little bit of time walking barefoot on the sand, watching the waves, and listening to the sound of the ocean before bed. As we were walking along the water's edge, a man made a comment about a piece of driftwood looking like an alligator, and we responded in a friendly manner. Next thing we knew, he was walking with us and telling us all about his life: his recent surgery, what he used to do for a living, what his eighty-year-old father used to do and is doing now, how his ex-wife destroyed his vehicle when they were divorcing ... on and on. We were polite, but eventually we disengaged, saying we needed to get back, and walked back the way we had come. It wasn't the evening on the beach I had envisioned, but at least the man was kind enough to give me a perfect example of oversharing.

If you feel this might be an issue for you, shift your focus to the other person. Have a mindset to understand rather than be understood. Listen to how deeply the other person is sharing and match that level of intimacy and detail. (It's not always easy; I catch myself frequently giving a long answer to a simple question.) Practice giving simple replies and only sharing more details if the other person asks more questions.

Always Shallow

I have a significant number of clients who come in frustrated that everyone they meet just seems to converse on a very shallow level. It makes me wish I could introduce those clients to one another.

There are plenty of social situations where it is appropriate to keep the conversation light, especially when you have no interest in getting to know the other person better. But if you want to develop a deeper relationship with someone, learn to ask good questions and give meaningful replies yourself. You can Google "good questions to ask in a conversation." It will turn up some great results. You will stand out if you learn to ask good questions and aren't afraid to answer them yourself.

> NOTE: Interested in learning more about having meaningful conversations? Human connection expert Lisa Kalfus has a passion for empowering authentic connections and deeper relationships. She empowers people to become masterful conversationalists by confidently going beyond the small talk to get closer, faster. I had the privilege of meeting her at a weekend wellness event hosted by good friends of mine, and she led all of us through an exercise in building deeper conversations (see Resources).

Not a Great Listener

Most people are not great listeners. We tend to be egocentric, as mentioned before. To be fair, though, most of us are never actively taught how to be a good listener or shown why it is so important. No matter the heart of the person listening, if the one sharing doesn't feel like they are being listened to, the relationship will never progress.

> NOTE: *I Hear You* by Michael S. Sorensen (mentioned earlier in Chapter 5) and *Be a Better Listener* by J.D. Obrice are two excellent books about listening. They are very different from each other, but they will both no doubt increase your skills and motivation to be a great listener (see Resources).

No Eye Contact

Do you have trouble making eye contact? Not looking someone in the eye can come from insecurity, shame, embarrassment, or discomfort. This is normal in some cultures, and we must be sensitive to that when we travel internationally. In most cultures, however, eye contact conveys connection. If you have trouble looking someone in the eye, it can make them wonder if you have something to hide. An insecure person might even wonder if they are so unattractive that it is uncomfortable to look at them. At the very least, it tends to create disconnection.

It is so reassuring to make eye contact. I'm not talking about a dead stare, of course. When you are talking, look at the person. Break eye contact for a moment and then come back while you are talking, and when someone else is talking, practice keeping eye contact. It conveys that you care and value the other person.

Distracted

Distraction could fit under the heading of not being a great listener, but the reality is that some people can balance distraction and listening. The problem is that the one who is sharing has a hard time knowing they are being heard. Even if the other party can prove they are listening, there is still a lack of care conveyed toward the person talking, and usually a great deal of aggravation is felt, even if they don't show it.

My husband and I are pretty tied to our devices. If we are sitting down, we are typically on our laptops or phones. We have a large capacity for accepting this in each other because we both do it, and we can typically listen to each other anyway.

I should have written that last paragraph in the past tense. We did this until we were exposed to *The Connection Codes* by Dr. Glenn and Phyllis Hill. I was blessed to attend a training by the Hills, where they demonstrated the value of giving your full attention to the other person in a conversation, along with the concept of "ooooing." To "oooo" is to make a sound that conveys you are present and listening. It can be an "mmmm," an "ahhh," an "ohhh," a "hmmm," or the like. You get the idea. In their book *The Connection Codes*, they explain that research shows "an audible response activates the brain of the person sharing, so audible is important (versus simply nodding or smiling)."

After sharing that training with my husband, we started working on putting down our devices when the other one was speaking and making direct eye contact. We also have gotten used to verbal acknowledgment when talking. We had resisted the world telling us we should do this, as we were both happy and content. We write our own marriage rules, and they work super well for us. But the Hills' training on the brain science of conversation convinced us to give it a try. When we started doing this, it felt good. In fact, it felt great!

Interrupting

I used to struggle with interrupting. I think sometimes my interrupting was just an enthusiastic response to what the other person was saying that bubbled out before they were completely finished. But other times, I think it came from getting bored with how long they took to say something. Other times, I am sure I thought what I had to share was more important. No doubt, it was sometimes because of the limits we had on our time together as well. Whatever my excuse, it was not a good feeling. That's not who I wanted to be.

This was a struggle for me until I had a good friend who was ten times worse than me at interrupting. When I was with her, I never got to finish a sentence, and she never seemed to notice. I know I can be long-winded, even verbose, and in that context, I can understand someone interrupting me. But that was not the case here. I couldn't even get a full thought out. I would go home so frustrated with all sorts of half thoughts in my head that were never completed. I was convinced God had put her in my life just to show me how terrible that habit is so I would be inspired to break it for good. I think it worked. It became an issue I gave myself grace for but could no longer tolerate.

I still catch myself interrupting from time to time, but I am happy to say I am much improved. I have myself pretty well convinced that I do care a lot more about what the other person has to say than hearing myself talk. That is key!

All of this is to say, if you are someone who constantly interrupts, that might prevent you from getting that next coffee invite. For me, it was more about choosing who I wanted to be. I wanted to be a person who valued others, and there is no better way to show that you value someone than to listen without interrupting. (This is such a valuable trait it just might get you a coffee date!)

Advice-Giving

I'll never forget what I learned about advice-giving from Kathy, whose home was one of over a thousand homes in the Redding area that burned to the ground in the Carr Fire. She told me that a great many people seemed to have advice for the people who were affected by the fire. She then went on to say, "You know, unsolicited advice is really just criticism." I remember being dumbfounded as I realized the truth in that statement.

After that, I always tried to ask if someone wanted my input on a matter they were sharing before jumping in to share my thoughts. If they said no, there was no reason to give anything except encouragement and support. In the rare instance that it was difficult to support someone's choice to decline my help, I found a simple "okay" with a nod worked.

Incessant advice-giving can ruin friendships. Julie shared that she had a good friend that she highly respected, but when they would get together to catch up on the latest happenings in their lives, her friend always had advice on whatever Julie shared. It got old quickly. Julie tried to clarify that she wasn't asking for advice and didn't want it, but her friend's behavior would only change for a short time. It took so much emotional energy to be with her that Julie finally had to start limiting her time with that friend.

If you find you have this tendency, I challenge you to give yourself grace and acceptance, and then, with compassionate curiosity, ask yourself, "What is driving my need to give advice?"

Boring

It's easy to get into a rut in life. You work a job, come home weary from the day, eat, maybe watch some television, and then retire for the night, just to do it all again tomorrow. This can be a real challenge for anyone who is retired and spending most of their time at home watching television. It is easy to eventually reach a place where you have nothing interesting to talk about. Unless your job is exciting or you have interesting hobbies, you can become a pretty boring person.

Some ideas to combat this include volunteering, reading, staying up to date on current events, exploring different topics of interest, traveling, going to museums and galleries, developing hobbies, or learning new skills. The pathway to being boring is usually gradual and comfortable. If you find this applies to you, be your own best friend and encourage yourself to take action. You may find your efforts attract some interesting people into your world!

Poor Hygiene

This may be obvious, but it is a truth nonetheless. Chronic body odor, bad breath, or other unpleasant smells associated with the body can make it difficult to be around someone. These issues are not always related to poor hygiene, but when medical conditions are the underlying cause, care and meticulous hygiene can go a long way. I understand that some cultures bathe less frequently and some people have less access to bathing. The point is to be aware of poor hygiene as a possible cause of social ostracization in some environments—especially among kids in school.

It is important to regularly bathe, wash your hair, use a nail brush to get underneath your fingernails, and brush your teeth. Check in with a good friend who will tell you the truth.

There is nothing wrong with you, but you may benefit from an upgrade! Enough said.

Always Accepting, Never Inviting

Ah, this was another fatal flaw of mine. I'm so thankful for friends who hung in there with me, making me feel wanted and all the while teaching me what being a good friend looks like: initiating get-togethers. I'm a bit of a loner, I run several businesses, and I tend to lose track of time. Those are my excuses, but they don't hold any water when it comes to making my friends feel appreciated and confident that I also cherish our friendship and desire their company. Ordinarily, people get tired of always being the one to initiate. I have been blessed with friends who were patient with me in this, and I am so grateful. Thanks to them, I am much improved.

You will see me mentioning this several times because it bears repeating. If you want to shorten a season of loneliness, don't wait for an invitation. Initiate. And if you are patient, you might even find a friend like me.

Never Offering Use of Your Home or Car

Similarly, another bad habit is never hosting at your home or offering your car for carpooling. I am happy to say I am much better at this one—at least until we moved into our condo and our space got much smaller. I'm still good about offering my car, though! As a former police officer, I typically prefer to drive anyway.

If you can't offer your home or car, then look for ways to make it up to the people who always do—like bringing the food or paying for gas. Maybe arrive early to help with preparations, or stay after the gathering to help clean up. Make sure your friends feel appreciated and not just taken advantage of!

Expecting Others to Always Work Around Your Schedule

Besides not being great at initiating, I was also not great at altering my schedule for friendships. It actually never crossed my mind—until God got ahold of me. Not everyone has the option to amend their working hours—in fact, few do—but in my case, it was because I tended to be a loner and ran several companies. I typically had my schedule all charted out in my mind. I had the flexibility to insert friendship time, but friendship time literally cost me money. It was hard to fit in. Again, I'm so grateful for the friends who have pursued me through the years. How did I wake up to my bad habit? I had an encounter with God Almighty in which He whispered in my ear, "Friendships require sacrifice."

Now, you might think I was a slow learner in this department, and no doubt I was (am). But when the Lord whispers something in your ear, it's a pretty big deal, so I pay attention. You've got to have some skin in the game, as they say. You don't have to sacrifice for acquaintances you consider friends, although it is nice when you can. But building covenant friendships, those enduring, family-like connections, demands a commitment of time and effort—and good friends deserve it.

Gossipy

How many times have I heard, "They talk about everybody else, so I'm sure they are talking about me"? It's a pretty good assumption. Everyone needs a good friend, mentor, or counselor with whom they can sort out relationship struggles, but even that should be done with humility and thoughtfulness. Having a mouth that runs on about everyone and everything does not build trust. In fact, it can cause avoidance. And no one wants that reputation. The Bible has some pretty strong words about gossip (see Romans 1:29–32, Proverbs 26:20–22).

> NOTE: Our church's senior leader, Bill Johnson, has a reputation for never speaking badly about another person. Someone asked him how he was able to do that, and with deep emotion, he replied, "I fear Jesus in them. I fear that I would speak badly about someone made in the image of God, someone that is so valued by God that Jesus died for them. I fear that I would portray them as something less valuable than that. I fear how God would deal with a person who would betray the people made in His image." That sums it up pretty well.

A Bible story that has greatly impacted me is in Genesis 9:20–23, when Noah's youngest son, Ham, finds his father drunk and naked in his tent and can't wait to run outside and tell his brothers. What is their response? His brothers, Shem and Japheth, take a blanket, walk backward, and cover up their father's nakedness while averting their eyes so that they won't see him naked. I love this story because it speaks to treating others with honor and protecting them even when their behavior may make for good gossip.

Being Negative/Critical

Pretty much everyone can relate to a time in their life when things felt pretty gloomy. In those seasons, it can be hard to see the positive side of anything. But weathering through a season of negativity is different from being stuck there. No one likes to be around a chronically negative person—except maybe other chronically negative people. A bad attitude, seeing the cup half empty all the time, can run people off faster than anything.

One of my favorite verses in the Bible is Philippians 4:8–9 (NLT), which says, "And now, dear brothers and sisters, one final thing. Fix your thoughts on what is true, and honorable, and right, and pure, and lovely, and admirable. Think about things that are excellent and worthy of praise. Keep putting into practice all you learned and received from me— everything you heard from me and saw me doing. Then the God of peace will be with you." If we all put this one passage into practice, this would be a very different world, wouldn't it?

But even putting it into practice for oneself can change one's internal world and relationships dramatically.

> NOTE: Struggling to take negative, critical thoughts captive? Try what I did. God showed me an imaginary gift box with a lid I could lift up. He showed me that I could capture any negative thought (see 2 Corinthians 10:5) and put it in that box mid-thought, put the lid back on top, and then redirect my thought to something positive—something that better reflected who I wanted to be and what I wanted to be thinking. It works! This has been a really helpful tool for me. With repetition, this trick also helps build new positive neural pathways in the brain while extinguishing the negative thought pathways.

A WORD OF ENCOURAGEMENT

Who do you like to be around? Be that person: thoughtful, kind, respectful, honoring, honest, and basically the opposite of everything listed in this chapter.

If you find yourself anywhere in the struggles mentioned in this chapter, like I did, take to heart this familiar saying: "Look for progress, not perfection." If you genuinely like someone and can convey that well in how you interact with them (without getting weird about it), I've found most people can't help but like you. They simply cannot resist. Will they want to hang around you and be your good friend? Well, that depends on many factors—many of which have nothing to do with you (see Section 1). So don't beat yourself up. Just keep to your journey of personal growth, loving people well along the way, and eventually, you will find your tribe, your people. Know that they are worth the effort and the wait.

If you find yourself overwhelmed by any of these issues and want support along the way, get help. A good therapist can help you get unstuck and bring fresh new insights that can be so helpful. We will discuss when to seek professional help in the next chapter.

CHAPTER 8

WHEN TO SEEK HELP

So how do you know when you need to get help? When I teach resiliency to disaster team volunteers, I always advise people to get help when whatever physical, emotional, or mental symptoms they are dealing with become a problem for them. There are many life factors that can affect the level of discouragement we feel in a season of loneliness. There may be more informing our experience than just being lonely. And sometimes, we need help sorting those things out.

Childhood wounds can affect how we feel about ourselves. They affect our self-talk, our self-worth, our identity, and even our ability to fight for ourselves and for a better life. Childhood trauma can leave us with shame and guilt. It can affect our attachment styles, making us either overly anxious for attachment or overly dismissive and avoidant—both responses serving as a form of emotional protection.

Experiences of rejection and abandonment, two of the deepest pains the human heart can feel, often leave us with severe anxiety. No one ever wants to feel the pain of rejection and abandonment again, and those experiences can make us afraid of getting into new relationships and losing existing ones.

Struggles with anxiety and depression or other experiences that get labeled as mental illness can greatly impact a person's resiliency as well. Physical conditions need to be ruled out, too. All of these add challenges to your internal world, and you can benefit from working with a caring doctor, therapist, counselor, and/or pastor.

OKAY, LET'S GET PRACTICAL!

It might be time to get help if you are struggling with any of the following:

Severe Depression

Sadness is healthy when we experience loss or disappointment, but it becomes problematic when we get stuck in that sadness. Our body can adjust to that "sad chemistry" and think that is our norm. It will do everything it can to keep us in that state. We've already covered a few solutions, but the challenge of depression is that it can make you not want to do anything.

It is important to recognize that depression has different levels of severity. With severe depression, it is hard to find any motivation at all. It can be hard even to get out of bed in the morning. Minimal daily functioning becomes an overwhelming challenge. Often, you can't get over depression on your own. It affects your self-care, your motivation, your energy, and your frame of mind.

You may need to pull a team together to help you get through it. A doctor, therapist, family member, friend, pastor, trainer, and coach can all encourage you to stay consistent with good self-care habits. Options that are known to help with depression include the following:

- a nutritious diet
- exercise
- sunshine
- supplementation
- bodywork, such as massages or body-focused trauma therapy
- far infrared light therapy
- cold plunge
- reading the Scriptures
- tools that challenge your thinking (such as Cognitive Behavioral Therapy, aka CBT)
- mindfulness

Sometimes medication is appropriate. If you feel you need it, make sure you are seeing a good doctor who knows what is best for you. You want a doctor who also recommends therapy and other life-giving practices, not one who just hands out prescriptions. I don't have a solid stance on the use of medication, but I've known many people who felt like it didn't help, many others who felt like it caused additional problems, and others still who quite literally couldn't function without it. Each person has to search out that world for themselves to see what works best for them.

Self-Imposed Extreme Isolation

Agoraphobia is when people develop a fear of leaving their home and getting into situations that will trigger a panic attack or leave them feeling trapped and unable to escape. If you struggle with this, you are not alone! Even celebrities experience agoraphobia, including Zac Efron, Kim Basinger, Barbra Streisand, Woody Allen, Donny Osmond, Emma Stone, and Sally Field.

Nowadays, with counseling available over video call, a person struggling with this issue can get help from their own home. Without treatment, agoraphobia can worsen and last for years. If you find it completely overwhelming to be in social settings to the extent that you isolate yourself at home, don't hesitate to seek help.

Debilitating Anxiety

Social anxiety disorder differs from agoraphobia in that the fear of having a panic attack in public doesn't stem from a concern about being trapped. The fear is more about rejection or embarrassment from being judged by others.

Generalized anxiety is characterized by persistent, excessive worry about things in everyday life, such as health, finances, and relationships. It causes irritability, sleeplessness, restlessness, and difficulty concentrating, and it can be very difficult to control.

Any time anxiety is affecting your freedom of movement and restricting your life, I recommend getting professional help. There are plenty of resources available (books, articles, podcasts, videos, etc.) on this topic that can increase your understanding, facilitate recovery, and supplement therapy as well.

> NOTE: I have compiled a short cheat sheet of different ways you can calm your nervous system and move from "fight or flight" into "rest and digest." You can find this list on my website (see Resources).

A Persistent Feeling of Loneliness All of One's Life

For some people, feeling lonely is all too familiar. When I ask my clients if they felt seen, heard, and understood as a child, it is the rare client that says yes. When I ask that question, it is not uncommon to see emotion well up in my client's face. I think that perhaps the most basic human need of all is to be seen, heard, understood, and valued. Unfortunately, even good parents are not always aware that caring for their children does not automatically convey this value to the child. It takes awareness, attention, and effort, and historically, that has not been taught to parents very well.

If you find yourself with no other reference to the experience of life than loneliness, I encourage you to seek out professional help. You are not defective. The right professional can help you find freedom. You were not born to be lonely all of your life.

Intrusive Thoughts or Repetitive Behaviors

Do you struggle with intrusive thoughts that make your mind feel like it is on a hamster wheel of sorts, going round and round with the same thoughts repeating over and over in your head? Do you feel helpless to control them? Or maybe you recognize familiar triggers that always set you off, causing you to lose control, and afterward you feel discouraged, embarrassed, and ashamed? Perhaps you are challenged with excessive, repetitive behaviors you can't control such as handwashing or checking to see if the front door is locked or the stove is turned off. If there is any area of your life where you feel stuck, I hope you know there are answers for you out there and people who are trained and ready to come alongside you and help. Don't hesitate to seek them out.

Driven by Only What Benefits You

Most of us know someone who is self-serving, thinks they know it all, listens to no one, is always defensive, shifts blame, and never admits they're wrong. They carry a sense of entitlement and seem to lack empathy. Of course, their awareness of being so is usually limited, if not nonexistent. Rarely do they see themselves as others do. If you recognize these traits in yourself, or if someone you love has been accusing you of these traits (people with this type of personality are most often the ones accusing others), give yourself grace and acceptance, then seek out professional help. Maybe it's you. Maybe it's them. Either way, this is probably the biggest relationship destroyer there is, so you will benefit from professional help.

Deep Despair, Suicidal Thoughts

Lastly, keep a mindful eye on yourself if you start feeling like life is not worth living or like you can't keep on as you have been. You would be surprised how many people have wrestled with these thoughts at some point in their lives. You are not alone. There is nothing wrong with you, but it is time to be your own best friend and put protections in place to keep yourself safe. Remove anything in your home that might put you at risk. There is no shame in it, but this is the time to get help on board. If there is no one in your life to whom you can stay accountable or call when you are in crisis, then seek professional help.

Suicide is incredibly destructive to families. As I mentioned before, I lost a cousin-in-law to suicide when I was seventeen. He was twenty-one. It was devastating. I've had other family members attempt to end their lives as well. Fortunately, by the grace of God, they were discovered in time for us to save them. I have friends who have also lost family members to suicide and several clients who lost a parent to suicide when they were young.

Jonas sought to end his life but was found in time. Afterward, he was profoundly impacted by the hurt he saw it had caused his family. For a long time after that, he struggled with wanting to end his life every day, but what kept him alive was thinking about the extreme emotional pain he had put his family through. He never wanted to hurt them like that again. That strength of will (and, no doubt, the prayers of family) kept him alive until he finally vanquished the desire to end his life. He is now living what I think he would call his best life. It was a struggle to get there, but he would tell you it was a battle worth fighting.

If you are feeling unsafe, don't be alone. Death is permanent and only dumps your problems on those you love and care about. Get help. Get a medical evaluation. Every single person I know who survived suicide was glad they did and found renewed hope for living.

A WORD OF ENCOURAGEMENT

The good news is that God has not left us without options to heal this pain in our hearts. Healing can come from a friend or family member, a coach, a teacher, a pastor, a mentor, and even a local support group or church community. In a season of loneliness, however, those may not be available or feel like enough. If you feel stuck or overwhelmed, or if you just want to heal faster, don't be afraid to seek out professional help.

> NOTE: Remember, sometimes we are fighting against more than flesh and blood (see Ephesians 6:12). There is usually a spiritual component at play. My church has a wonderful deliverance ministry called Sozo, and there are many similar ministries around the world. There are so many testimonies of breakthrough and freedom that come from these ministries. You can check out what our center offers in the way of counseling or Sozo with both in-person and video appointments on the Transformation Center website listed in the Resources section at the end of this book.

God's desire for you is a life of peace and joy. He is so passionate about you being free and healed that He has given us many different ways to facilitate healing. Don't be afraid to pursue help. There are a variety of healing modalities that different specialists, therapists, and counselors use. I have mentioned a few in this book, but there are many more. You don't have to stay stuck, and you don't have to go on this journey alone.

We've looked quite extensively at why loneliness is so pervasive in our world. We've also looked at things you can do to thrive and build community in a season of loneliness. But perhaps you're reading this book because someone you love is struggling with loneliness. In the next section, we'll discuss ideas for helping to address the unique needs of kids (Chapter 9) and the elderly (Chapter 10).

SECTION 4

LOVED ONES

HELPING THOSE YOU LOVE THRIVE

SECTION 4 INTRODUCTION

WHEN YOU ARE CONCERNED FOR SOMEONE ELSE

Perhaps you picked up this book not for yourself but for someone you love. If you have a friend struggling with loneliness, hopefully the prior chapters will be a help to you in supporting them. If you love a child or elderly person struggling with loneliness, this section offers unique ways to help them. Loneliness and the pain and sadness that come with it are very real experiences, and it can be hard to watch someone you love struggle with these feelings. I felt it was important to address these particular age groups because they both have special needs.

The same basic tenets mentioned so far in this book are important for a child or older person to understand. They need to know there is nothing wrong with them and that loneliness does not have to be a forever state. However, because of the limitations inherent to these age groups, children and the elderly may need you to be proactive on their behalf.

If you know someone older or younger struggling with loneliness, I hope that this last section will be helpful. May it give you ideas and spur new thoughts about how you can offer help.

CHAPTER 9

HOW TO HELP YOUR LONELY CHILD

Special Thoughts for Kids and Teens

Experiencing loneliness can be crushing for anyone. To watch your child struggling with loneliness can be excruciating—especially if you wrestled with loneliness as a child yourself. The pain is all too real.

Young children can experience loneliness when they move to a new neighborhood or school, especially if they are shy. Incidences of prejudice and bullying are far more common than anyone would wish. If a child feels ashamed or embarrassed about getting bullied, they may be hesitant to tell anyone, especially if they think it will only make the bullying worse.

If a child has a health condition or disability that requires special accommodations, they may feel different or be teased about it and end up isolating.

Similarly, if a child comes from another country, experiencing cultural changes and learning a new language may be overwhelming and present challenges in interacting with their peers. They may find it easier to simply withdraw.

Changes in the home, such as a new baby, a parent changing jobs, divorce, or a newly blended family, can affect a child at school as well. If a child feels lonely or abandoned at home, they will often carry a diminished perspective of themselves to school.

When a teenager is struggling with loneliness, it can be scary for a parent. The teenage years can be rough for so many reasons, and emotions are typically heightened during this life stage. Teenagers often live in the extremes of "always" and "never." This can lead to greater despair if they are also struggling with loneliness. All the challenges that lend themselves to loneliness in both children and adults can be experienced by teenagers, and their coping skills are not yet fully developed.

In addition, teenagers feel more pressure regarding academics and what they will do once they graduate from high school. High school is when young adults are typically expected to figure out who they are. Friend groups are ever-changing.

Cliques are common. The "in crowd" and the "out crowd" are common descriptors of how teenagers perceive their classmates. If they are struggling with loneliness, most likely they will see themselves as being a part of the out crowd—or maybe entirely invisible.

Mental health issues are sometimes noticed for the first time in the teenage years, complicating just about everything. Issues related to sexuality, gender, abuse, racism, drugs, and alcohol also come into play. Overall, it's not an easy time.

I don't think anything is harder on the heart of a parent than watching their child suffer. Many parents will be tempted to rescue their child in an attempt to spare them pain, and sometimes there is a place for this sentiment. We are certainly called to protect our children from abuse and danger. But more often than not, as they get older, the best way we can serve our children through the challenges of growing up, like loneliness, is by coming alongside them, offering them guidance and support, encouraging them, and expressing our belief that they will prevail. This is the best way we can prepare our children for life: by helping them learn how to navigate hard times.

> NOTE: Interested in some great parenting resources? Check out Brittney and Ben Serpell's Loving on Purpose website, Brittney's book Imperfect Parenting, and their podcast *Imperfect Parenting*, where they share ways for parents to cultivate a loving, heart-to-heart connection with their children (see Resources).

OKAY, LET'S GET PRACTICAL!

HOW YOU CAN HELP:

Be Available

The best gift we can give our children is availability. This should be established when they are young, but it is never too late. Being available means giving your child face time. It means listening and meeting their need to feel seen and heard, understood and valued. This can be especially challenging with teenagers, who are known for not being ready to talk when parents are. It's a special parent who will miss out on sleep to talk to their teen late at night, but the gift to your child and your relationship is priceless.

Children do not keep us from what is important. If you have kids, they are what is important.

Surely sometimes children can benefit from learning to wait. They should learn manners, such as not interrupting, but some of these lessons come with age. Setting the stage for your child to know you are always there for them, that you care about their experience and are ready to help them through it, starts at birth. This is important in every season of a child's life, but especially when they are struggling with loneliness. When they are wondering if anyone cares, if anyone likes them, they must know you do. Show you care by being available with compassion and a listening ear.

Be Nonjudgmental

This can be tough because we, as parents, want to train our children in the values and beliefs we hold dear. Still, it is important to realize that helping a child navigate core values in life comes best with understanding, not with criticism and judgment.

When I was in the police force, I had a keen sense that we were not the ones in charge of punishment. That was the court's job. I worked for an excellent police department and had the privilege of working with great officers, but I noticed that, at times, some of my fellow officers didn't have that same perspective. I would watch them verbally shame people who were caught breaking the law. I think there is a natural tendency in us to believe we can shame someone out of a behavior, but it doesn't work that way. We are much more likely to behave in a way that matches who we believe we are, and when we receive messages of shame, all too often we take on that shame as part of our identity, and we continue to act it out. You don't want to do that to your kids. Their self-talk will mirror how you talk to them.

Having been a therapist who studied human behavior, I came into law enforcement knowing that anyone breaking the law has a history that explains why they are where they are.

I always felt it was only by the grace of God that I was in the front seat and they were in the back. No one grows up with the life goal of being hauled off in the backseat of a police car and going to jail.

My experience helped me to speak with many of the people I arrested adult-to-adult (sometimes adult-to-kid). I knew that being arrested was humiliating. Having a spotlight thrown on your struggles is embarrassing. I found that when I treated them with respect, listened, and shared my perspective without judgment, they frequently took responsibility for their actions and were ready to deal with the consequences and move on.

It is the same with kids struggling with loneliness—the experience is embarrassing and painful. If you can be present and come alongside them, without berating or shaming, your child will be much more open to sharing their struggles with you. Sometimes, people want so badly to be liked by their child that they will abdicate being the parent, choosing to be more of a friend. This often results in a poor outcome for the child. In this case, however, being your child's friend is being a good parent.

WHAT YOU CAN TEACH:

Teach Your Child How to Manage Their Inner Dialogue

Remember the tools I shared in Section 2? Here is a quick review:

1. Listen to how you talk to yourself.

2. Take a stance of compassionate curiosity.

3. Acknowledge your feelings.

4. Give yourself grace and acceptance.

Learn and practice these yourself, and you will be able to teach your child how to do the same.

A season of loneliness can breed a lot of negative self-talk and even self-hatred. When the pain is too much, a child may shut down their feelings. Teaching your child these tools will preemptively help buffer them in a season of loneliness. However, if you find yourself reading this while your child is already struggling, know that it is not too late for them to benefit from these techniques. This time can provide a good opportunity for your child to become aware of their inner dialogue and learn how to manage it. If they can start learning this practice in childhood, it will benefit them for the rest of their life.

Teach Your Child Values

It is surprising how many of my clients had to figure out life on their own. Now, as adults, they come to therapy questioning their choices and thoughts on a variety of issues. I love these clients! They are always such great people. Some come from terrible homes, but many just come from busy homes—homes where they were taught values around *doing* things, like taking a bath, doing their homework, and cleaning their plate, but with little awareness or attention given to their inner world and establishing core values to live by. Too often, parents leave this training to the school or church, only to be frustrated when this doesn't play out as they had hoped.

Often, when children feel lonely, they may be tempted to compromise their values in an attempt to be accepted by their peers. We see this so often with teenagers. Again, it pays to be preemptive and address this topic early on by teaching your child how important it is to maintain good core values, no matter the circumstance they find themselves in. Core values are foundational to who we are as people. They are a part of our identity. The stronger your child's sense of self, the better they will weather the challenges of loneliness. Just as with the tools mentioned above, if you are reading this because your child is already struggling with loneliness, take heart. This can be a valuable time to connect as a parent and give your child that one-on-one attention, pouring into their identity and helping them establish who they want to be with plenty of affirmation and encouragement.

Teach Your Child Good Social Skills

Have you ever been around someone who interrupts all the time? No one wants to be around that person. Teach your child how to truly listen when someone talks. Teach them about eye contact, attentive facial expressions, and verbal responses. Show them how to ask open-ended questions, how to wait for someone to finish speaking, and how to put more importance on what the other person is sharing than on what they themselves want to say. These are good skills for anyone to learn and improve upon, but teaching good social skills to a child who is lonely can go a long way toward helping them overcome their struggles.

Teach Your Child How to Be a Good Friend

Don't assume your child knows what it takes to be a good friend. Think about what makes a person a good friend and teach these traits to your child. Kindness, thoughtfulness, empathy, humility, encouragement, courage, honesty, generosity, and gratitude are a few I highly value.

> NOTE: I'm reminded of Galatians 5:22–23 (NLT): "But the Holy Spirit produces this kind of fruit in our lives: love, joy, peace, patience, kindness, goodness, faithfulness, gentleness, and self-control. There is no law against these things!" That's a good list to keep in mind!

Additionally, when your child feels loved—seen, heard, understood, and valued—they will know how to love and value others well. Loving your child well and actively modeling these behaviors for them goes a long way, but it's also worth talking about these values and teaching them, rather than expecting them to be acquired through assimilation.

Additionally, when you teach your child how to be a good friend, you are also teaching them what to expect from their friends. This will raise their awareness and, hopefully, prevent them from rushing into unhealthy friendships just to relieve the pain of loneliness.

ACTIONS YOU CAN TAKE:

Facilitate Friendships

Open your home to your child's friends. Host parties and sleepovers. Be a fun place for kids to hang out. If that isn't workable for your situation, plan playdates. Get to know their friends' parents. Offer to babysit. Offer to carpool. Sign your child up for activities and classes outside of school (e.g., sports, gymnastics, dance, art) and be involved enough to help your child develop those relationships. I took private art lessons during elementary school, and the friendships formed in that early art class have lasted a lifetime!

I realize some of these ideas can be extra challenging to a single parent or a family on a tight budget, but if you fall into one or both categories, you are used to the challenge of finding creative solutions. What could you do to facilitate friendships in a way that costs minimal time and money?

Help Your Child Develop into an Interesting Person

Giving your child different experiences not only brings potential friends into their world but also gives them bandwidth for connecting with a lot of different people throughout their life. Shared interests and experiences connect us. Your child's experiences will make them interesting, provide topics of conversation, and build their self-confidence, both in the present and later in life.

—*Collections* are another good way to connect your child with others—even when they are built at home. I collected coins when I was a child. My sister collected stamps. It's amazing how many times my coin collection has come up in conversations as an adult. Set your kid up for social success. Teach them the fun and wonder that comes with collecting.

—*Look for activities and clubs* that might pair well with your child's interests. I'm not an advocate for having a child sign up for every activity and sport available. I'm a big believer that kids need downtime as much as or more than we do, but having some outside activities can be great for cultivating friendships. Common examples, both in and outside of school, are gymnastics, dance lessons, art classes, science groups, choir, band, orchestra, cheerleading, pep squad, drama, chess club, language clubs, and sports.

—*Classes in the community* can provide a fun opportunity for parent and child to create together. As mentioned in Chapter 5, most communities offer a variety of classes. Craft stores, libraries, community colleges, and universities will typically post a calendar for their classes online. Many of the community classes offered are suitable for or specifically designed for kids. My friends Dan and Nancy Barrett have started a nonprofit, Until Now Creative, in Wenatchee, Washington, that provides a variety of creative art classes for people of all ages, kids included (see Resources). I wish I lived closer; it looks like great fun!

—*Youth groups offered by local churches* should not be overlooked as opportunities for combating loneliness and developing friendships. My closest friends growing up were friends I made in a youth group. Our parents knew each other, and we shared common values and beliefs. I have so many wonderful memories of being in these friends' homes, roaming all over town on our bikes, and going to various out-of-town activities by bus or caravan. There were times when I felt celebrated in these homes in a way I wasn't in my own home, and that can go a long way in keeping a kid encouraged in life.

Schools will also often allow outside groups to host Christian clubs on campus. Fellowship of Christian Athletes is one example I know of.

—*Homeschooling activities* can present challenges when it comes to forming friendships. I've had clients who were homeschooled and grew up with their siblings being their only friends. Fortunately, I think this is the exception. The homeschooling movement has grown so much in the last few decades that now there are plenty of opportunities to connect with other homeschool families and build friendships outside the home. As kids get exposed to different personalities and different families' ways of living, these outside activities can become a valuable and necessary component of a child's social development.

Volunteer Together

Every church and every community has volunteer opportunities. By volunteering together, you not only model serving others to your child and create special family memories, but you also open the opportunity for them to make new friends. These types of shared experiences readily provide their own conversation material and can make new connections much easier. And in the meantime, you and your child are providing benefit to your church or community and helping to build a healthy self-image in your child in the process. Serving others almost always makes us feel good about ourselves. Feeling good about themselves will go a long way in helping your child weather the ups and downs of friendship that can sometimes result in a lonely season.

WHAT TO DO IF EXTRA HELP IS NEEDED:

Seek Professional Support

This bears repeating: Don't hesitate to get the help of a professional therapist, counselor, coach, mentor, or pastor for your child. Sometimes, another adult can step in and help in a way parents cannot. A good therapist can give your child tools that will improve their ability to feel good about themselves and to connect well with others.

A WORD OF ENCOURAGEMENT

Don't lose heart! Your kids are experiencing life! And while they are still in your home, you have the opportunity to help them walk through some of life's challenges. Your child's season of loneliness can be an opportunity for the two of you to get to know each other better. It is an opportunity to foster a closer connection and impart values, to instill belief in themselves, and to have fun together as a family while you still have a bird's-eye view into their day-to-day world.

None of us parent perfectly—many of us wish for a do-over. But if you can show your child how to navigate life with its many ups and downs, you're doing well. Giving them the skills they need will equip them to face the challenges that inevitably come in life. Don't get lost in your child's despair. Come alongside them and turn this season of loneliness into one of opportunity.

I'll end with one of my favorite verses—a promise for our children:

> "I will teach all your children,
> and they will enjoy great peace."
>
> —Isaiah 54:13 (NLT)

CHAPTER 10

HOW TO HELP YOUR LONELY AGING PARENTS

Strategies for Families Both Close and Far Away

I'm not sure anything in life truly prepares you for caring for elderly parents—unless you got to witness your parents or a friend doing so. The challenges, if you live nearby, can be overwhelming. If you live long-distance, you are spared some of the daily responsibilities, but the distance can greatly exacerbate the challenge of trying to provide your parent(s) with good care.

What is the saying? "Growing old is not for sissies!" So true. After I left home, my dad's mother moved from Ponca City, Oklahoma, the town she had lived in for most of her adult life, to an apartment forty miles away in Stillwater, Oklahoma, where my parents lived. I can remember her telling me that everyone she knew was dead. My grandfather had died some ten years earlier, and she had outlived all her friends. That struck me as so profound. I had always intended to live a long life. I had not considered all the goodbyes that might be involved if I succeeded. My grandmother was eighty-one when she died.

In contrast, my mother's father lived to be ninety-seven. He lived in a retirement home, was active at church, and became known as quite the pool shark in the retirement community. He had a lot of friends, making new ones all along the way. He outlived two wives and married for a third time in his eighties. After the death of my fifteen-year-old daughter, he encouraged me to look at life as an adventure. I think it was the only advice he ever gave me, but it was a jewel. Certainly, no matter our circumstances, life is what we make it, and perspective is everything.

I was making the final edits on this manuscript when my mom died. Though she was approaching her ninety-first birthday and battling dementia, her death came suddenly and unexpectedly. I had to go back through the book and change every mention of my mom to the past tense. That was sobering and a little surreal.

My mom was living in an assisted living facility in Edmond, Oklahoma. She made the decision to sell her home and move into a retirement center six months after my dad died. She eventually had to be moved to assisted living as her health and mind started declining. Her younger sister, herself in her eighties, lived in town and visited her every day, and that was a tremendous help. Two of my siblings lived within driving distance, one an hour away and one four hours away, which was also helpful. My youngest brother and I, meanwhile, were pretty far away, both of us living in California. My mom was not interested in moving, so we were faced with loving her from a distance—extra challenging for all of us as dementia set in.

Having an elderly mom living in an assisted living facility made this chapter deeply personal to me from the outset. Realizing that the things I share here literally affect the last years of our family members' lives makes it all the more personal. I hope some of these ideas will provide you with some great activities to make those years enjoyable for your loved one. Obviously, what you can do to help your parent(s) is going to depend on many factors. My hope here is to give you some sparks that will spur ideas of your own—whether you live in the same town as your parent(s) or some distance away.

OKAY, LET'S GET PRACTICAL!

Many of these ideas came from the American Association of Retired Persons (AARP). I found them to be a great resource for ideas on a variety of topics directed toward older people.

I've added to the list and divided it into two sections: one for parents in the same town and one for long-distance parents. You will see that some ideas are meant to connect you with your parent(s) to aid in preventing their loneliness, while other ideas are for connecting them with other people. There is also a great deal of overlap. Additionally, I will refer to these family members as parents, but what is shared here certainly applies to grandparents, aunts, uncles, and any other older family member.

IDEAS FOR FAMILY MEMBERS WHO LIVE CLOSE:

If you live in the same town, there is an endless list of things you can do to help a lonely parent, depending on their level of functioning. If your parent lives in a residential facility, it may offer activities you can do together with your parent. If I visited on the right night, my mom would rope me into going down and playing bingo with them. It was a lot of fun, and we would both go back to her room with a handful of diet-ruining candy bars we had won. Her facility frequently had entertainment come in and perform in the shared living area. Meals were provided in either a dining room or her private room. Guests were usually welcome to join family members (for an additional fee). Churches came in and provided worship services and communion. Her facility even allowed pets.

Watch Television Together

My mom loved the game show channel, and she left it playing all day long. When I visited, we would make a game of it and play along. Sometimes, I was the only one playing along, since she had dozed off a good bit, but I knew she enjoyed the company.

Do Jigsaw Puzzles Together

When I went to see my mom, there was always a puzzle in progress somewhere in the facility. My mom didn't like puzzles very much, but others in her community really enjoyed them. My ninety-seven-year-old aunt from my dad's side of the family lived in that same facility. She and I had a great time sitting at the puzzle table together, helping each other hunt for the piece to fill that spot we both had our eye on. If you have extra puzzles around your home, think about sending them to your parent or to a local retirement home. (Now as I send my book off for its final proofing, I'm sad to report that my aunt just passed away early this morning.)

Get Them a Pet

As mentioned earlier, research has shown that a lot of health benefits can come from owning a pet. For elderly parents in particular, not only can pets help with loneliness, but they have been shown to improve recovery after a heart attack or stroke, as well as possibly extend life expectancy. Pets that are entertaining yet fairly easy to care for include any animal in a cage or aquarium, such as fish, reptiles, or birds. Dogs and cats are always popular and easy to love, so long as parents have assistance or the ability to give their pets the extra attention they need.

Help with Social Media

If your parent is fairly capable with technology, you can help them set up a social media account. If they have an account but have lost the ability to navigate the platform on their own, plan a coffee date now and then during which you can browse through their page and their friends' pages together. This can be especially meaningful around their birthday or on holidays.

Go on Field Trips

If your parent is able to get out, taking them on a daytime adventure can do wonders for their spirits. Once, when I was in town, a friend and I took my mom on an outing to the National Cowboy and Western Heritage Museum in Oklahoma City (known as the Cowboy Hall of Fame when I was growing up). We put her in a wheelchair provided by the museum. It was great fun and made for a great memory.

LONG-DISTANCE IDEAS (THAT WORK LOCALLY AS WELL):

Send Cards and Letters

It is almost a lost art, but receiving a card with a handwritten note or a handwritten letter in the mail is still a treat to most people. Many older adults eventually lose their ability to use the electronic devices they once were familiar with, and emails can get buried pretty fast. A card or letter is something they can hold on to and keep close by to read again and again if they like. If their memory is failing, including a photo of yourself may help them associate the card with you.

Engage Delivery Services

If your parent still lives in their home, you can have a meal sent by a meal delivery service like GrubHub or DoorDash. Some communities have Meals on Wheels, which personally delivers prepared meals to the homes of older adults. These volunteers are typically wonderful about stopping in and chatting for a few moments when they deliver. Every older adult I know who gets meals delivered by Meals on Wheels looks forward to their delivery person stopping in for a few minutes. These services have the added benefit of helping your parent get good nutrition.

Delivery of groceries using services like Instacart can also foster relationships. I have friends who work for Instacart, and they have clients who request them regularly because they like them and the choices they make for them in the stores.

Some pharmacies have delivery services. My husband and I used to run and get prescriptions for our elderly neighbor before she passed away. I know delivering them always included a little bit of a visit.

You may find an errand-running service in your parents' community that can fill many gaps and includes a little bit of conversation with the customers in their service. (That could be a great business to start as well.) All these services can bring more people into a parent's otherwise lonely world.

Hire Help

Even in assisted living, my mom would have loved having someone to sit with her full-time every day just to keep her company. There were times when she needed extra assistance in her apartment. That level of care is very expensive, but thankfully, my dad left her well cared for, so it wasn't an issue.

Hiring someone to come in and clean a parent's home not only keeps their living environment clean but also provides a regular visit from someone. This service was included in what my mom paid for her apartment, but if your parent is still in their home, it won't be. My mom also had a beautician she could go to who had a shop within the facility. If your parent is still in their home, sometimes you can find a traveling beautician who will do house calls. We also have a mobile vet in our community, which can be helpful if your parent has a pet.

Friendly relationships can be built when the help is at least weekly, so if you have the financial resources, this is a great way to help a lonely parent.

Watch Shows, Documentaries, and Movies Apart but Together

This can take a little finessing, but whether you're streaming or watching regular television, it can be fun to "watch a show together" and talk about it afterward. One of you can turn off your television's volume, or you can mute each other and then unmute to talk.

Make Phone Calls and Video Calls

This is easier if your parent can still use their smartphone, tablet, or computer. Services like Zoom, FaceTime, and Skype are great because they allow you to see each other while you talk. Seeing one another bridges the distance and gives more of a feeling of being together. If your parent struggles with these apps, they may need to enlist help.

If conversation is hard, you can read them a book or play them an audiobook from a service like Audible or Chirp. Local libraries often have loanable audiobook services, too. (As mentioned, check out the Libby or Hoopla apps.)

Some people even manage to play board games over a video call. This can be fun for grandkids but definitely requires some savvy on both sides. A game like bingo is probably the simplest idea.

You can also sing to them, sing together, or listen to music over the phone together. For a special occasion, you could record a short video of yourself playing an instrument or singing and send it to your parent. That would give them something special to watch over and over.

Another video call idea is to reach out to family members or a longtime friend of your parent and coordinate a group call. Zoom works great for this, but other options include Google Meet and Microsoft Teams.

Assemble and Send an Activity Box

Base what you put in the activity box on your parent's interests. Do they like crossword puzzle books or jigsaw puzzles? Sudoku? Do they crochet or knit? Adult coloring books have become very popular. You can even add nice gifts, like a candle, lotion, or a handkerchief.

Help Your Parent Get Connected in the Community

Many communities have a senior center that hosts activities geared toward the elderly. They are also a good source of information about resources in the community. If transportation is an issue, check and see if the community offers a senior or special needs transportation service. If a parent is mobile, getting out can immensely alleviate the isolation they feel.

Help Them Find Purpose and Fulfillment

As you get older, it is easy to feel like you are simply existing, that you have lived past your purpose or ability to give something to the world. I saw my mom's dwindling sense of purpose be reignited when she joined a group that crocheted little stocking caps for the local hospital's newborn nursery. When I went to visit, she proudly showed me all of the hats she had made that were waiting to get picked up. It made such a difference in her demeanor and connected her to others in the group. I genuinely felt her loss and saw her sense of purpose deflate again when the group was told the hospital had enough caps and didn't need more.

Another older woman I knew had a card-writing ministry. Every now and then, I would be the recipient of one of her cards. It was usually filled with encouragement and sometimes a Scripture. I always thought she was doing such a beautiful service. I didn't know anyone else doing something like that. Some groups sponsor letter writing to service men and women in active duty. Some churches have a ministry for writing letters to prisons. And every missionary I know (and I know a lot) would love to get a card from someone, to know someone is thinking of and praying for them.

Sometimes, our parents need a little help from us to figure out what they can do that will make a contribution and feel meaningful to them.

Maybe your parent would enjoy sponsoring a child through an organization such as World Vision or Compassion International. Most of these organizations also facilitate regular correspondence of photos and letters from the sponsored child to their sponsor, so with the sense of fulfillment from helping a child also comes connection.

Encourage Them to Explore New Interests

It's easy to fall into a rut of familiarity in life—especially as we get older. Is there something that would bring a new spark of interest to your parent? If they have a chair with a view out a window, you might consider setting up a bird feeder directly on the window or outside on a post. We get a monthly delivery of "no-waste bird seed" from Amazon and enjoy watching the birds outside on our patio. Depending on your parent's abilities or available assistance, other ideas they may like include scrapbooking, filling out a memory book, or painting.

Hire a Professional Listening Service

During the pandemic, my mom was shut in her apartment. They delivered her meals to her door, and she had very little contact with anyone for months. We saw this isolation significantly affect her morale and cognitive functioning. It was during the pandemic that the idea of starting a professional listening service came to me. At the time, I had never heard of such a service, but now there are several of them. I named my company A Listening Friend (see Resources). If you are unable to talk to your parent as much as you would like, let a listening service fill that gap.

A WORD OF ENCOURAGEMENT

Everyone's parents are in different circumstances. Some may be in their own home. Others may be in a care facility. Some parents can still drive and get around. Others are more restricted in their mobility. Some parents are able to get out and get involved in activities, while other parents will need some creative solutions that can come to them.

It is hard caring for a lonely parent with an abundance of time on their hands when your own world is busy. A little bit of creative thought and effort can go a long way in bettering their world—and helping you feel better about yourself as their son or daughter. Give yourself grace. Caring for aging parents presents a lot of challenges. We haven't even discussed issues like dementia, terminal illness, personality challenges, and childhood wounds, but these are subjects for a more complex book. My hope here is to give you a few ideas of things you might be able to do if you want to help your parent. There are a lot of factors that are out of your control, but anything you can do to show you care will go a long way in facilitating your parent's well-being.

THE CONCLUSION
AND MORE

CONCLUSION

IS THIS FOREVER?

Is loneliness forever? The answer is no. A season of loneliness, no matter how extended it may be, will pass if you are proactive and don't give up. Often, it will resolve itself, but *you must be a willing participant*. It requires courage and patience. It requires a willingness to grow and not shrink back, to deal with fears and patterns of thinking and behaving that don't serve you. If you commit to growth, I promise you will like who you become in the process!

The time you are in right now may be your "valley of the shadow of death" (Psalm 23:4) or, as one of my church's pastors, Kris Vallotton, would say, your "hell in the hallway." It is that uncomfortable stretching place between where you were and where you are going. It's the required place of testing before you reach the door of your destiny, that place where the Enemy will do all he can to steal, kill, and destroy your future happiness (John 10:10). But it's important to remember that this is a challenge to get *through*, not trapped in. Partner with growth, partner with encouragement, partner with God. Get whatever help you need so that you don't get stuck.

Don't lose hope, and don't quit. It will be worth it in the end!

A WORD OF ENCOURAGEMENT

If you find yourself in a season of loneliness, know that you are not alone. Over a third of the world is struggling with loneliness, with some surveys reporting as high as two-thirds. There are so many factors that may be contributing, but none of them has the power to keep you lonely forever. No matter how long your season has been, you can break free. This is not your plight in life. It is a matter of finding the answers that are out there. So many have gone ahead of you and won this battle. It is my sincerest hope that this book will serve to help you on your own journey to find joy and build community.

FINAL THOUGHTS FROM MY HEART

The thoughts I want to share here are not for everyone. If you are in pain from loneliness, please know that matters, and it is important to pay attention to that pain and the thoughts and emotions underneath it. Pushing pain down or away sometimes helps in the moment, but it is never a good long-term solution. What I share here in these final words is not meant to drive you to push the pain away because of shame or guilt. It is meant as a spiritual solution, a ladder out of the mire, out of what can be a bottomless pit of self-pity and loneliness. If you are not looking for a spiritual solution, hopefully you will find something helpful to you in the earlier chapters of this book.

For Those Who Don't Know Jesus

If you don't know Jesus, your life will be transformed by meeting Him. He is God, who came to the earth as the Son of God, who lived as a man like us, and who now lives eternal. He is still personally available to you through His Holy Spirit. Ask Him to reveal Himself to you and keep all your senses open to experience Him. He is faithful to reveal Himself. He might do it immediately, or He might require you to seek Him out. He is safe, and you can trust Him. He is the source of so much wisdom and comfort. Jeremiah 29:13 (NIV) says, "You will seek me and find me when you seek me with all your heart."

Another verse I love in the Old Testament of the Bible is Isaiah 41:13 (NLT), which says, "For I hold you by your right hand—I, the Lord your God. And I say to you, 'Don't be afraid. I am here to help you.'"

Invite Jesus in as Lord of your life, and your life will never be the same.

For Those Who Know Jesus

Loneliness is a very real experience. I think Jesus must have experienced it as well, though He shares in John 16:32 that even when He was abandoned by all His followers, He was not entirely alone because He knew the Father was always with Him. He is always with you too. Following Jesus doesn't solve all our problems. In fact, He assured us that our lives would be full of trials and sorrow in the very next verse: "I have told you all this so that you may have peace in Me. Here on earth you will have many trials and sorrows. But take heart, because I have overcome the world" (John 16:33, NLT).

What does that mean, that He has "overcome the world?" It means that we can have victory through Him.

The question is, how do we access that victory? I believe there are always practical ways God gives us to access victory, and I have shared some of those ways in this book.

But there are also spiritual mindset issues that often come into play.

People want life to look a certain way. When it doesn't, a whole slew of emotions, discouragement, and doubts flood their thoughts and their heart. I know this from working with many people in crisis. It often affects their connection to God. The tendency can be to turn away from Him rather than toward Him. *The best advice I could ever give anyone is to keep your face turned toward Him, no matter what.*

True freedom comes from having a bigger picture of our life, recognizing what we live for. Sure, there are things I'd like to have or to change. But I also surrender them to the bigger picture of what my life is about, and that is a life lived for Him—praising Him, worshiping Him, being devoted to Him, surrendering to Him. Surrender means I will give up my anger, sadness, and pain about the disappointments in my life and release my life story to Him. It means I will praise Him no matter my circumstances.

(Don't think I have this down perfectly. I, like you, am a work in progress, but this is how I position my heart for what is truly important to me. Admittedly, it sometimes requires more wrestling with my flesh than I would like.)

I had another encounter with the Lord I will share here in hopes that it will give meaning to your life right where you are.

I was ministering to a woman who had been caring for her mother in her mother's home for a long time. She was very discouraged as she saw no short-term end to her situation, and all the plans and dreams she had for her life were on hold. She felt she was just watching her life go by, with all her gifts and talents going to waste.

As I ministered to her, God took me into an encounter of His perspective. He showed me that when we honor Him even when we don't understand why our circumstances are what they are—when we choose to worship Him in the midst of our confusion and disappointment—a very special fragrance comes off of that worship. It is a fragrance that only comes out of surrendered worship. It is a gift given out of pain that bears such a precious fragrance, a special incense, that rises to the heavens, and it cannot be offered once our circumstances change. He told me that when we do this, it places a table *before Him* in the presence of *His enemy* (as Psalm 23 says He does for us)! And then He said to me, "What greater way could someone spend their life?"

The Lord asked that question in a way that profoundly answered it, and it deeply impacted me. I experienced the awe of God in that moment. All of a sudden, every earthly achievement paled in comparison. I learned that even in the midst of our dreams not coming true, none of our plans working out, our prayers feeling unanswered, and God feeling far away, we still have the unique opportunity to step into what God said, and that was the highest calling.

As a final word, if you are struggling through the pain of loneliness—or any other discouraging life challenge—know that you have an opportunity right now to offer Him this uniquely fragrant gift of adoration and honor. You have the ability to set a table before God Almighty in the presence of His enemy. As you apply the principles in this book, in the very midst of the struggle, don't pass up this opportunity.

May God bless you on this journey.

Leslie

Be encouraged.
Be proactive.
Don't quit.
Keep your face toward God.

NEXT STEPS

Ways you can work with me:

Work with me as a pastoral therapist through the Bethel Transformation Center: https://www.betheltransformationcenter.com.

Work with me or a member of my team as a listener for conversation without advice or counsel through A Listening Friend: https://www.alisteningfriend.com.

Work with me as a personal or corporate consultant, personal life coach, or speaker: leslieparkertaylor@gmail.com.

AND ... HOW YOU CAN HELP!

Could you take two minutes now to leave a helpful review on Amazon, sharing what you thought of this book? I created this link to make it quick and easy: OvercomingLonelinessReview.com.

Thank You!

RESOURCES

Christian Counseling Center and Inner Healing Ministry
- Bethel Transformation Center—www.betheltransformationcenter.com

Professional Listening Service
- A Listening Friend—www.alisteningfriend.com

Books Referenced
- *Anatomy of an Illness: As Perceived by the Patient* by Norman Cousins
- *Atomic Habits* by James Clear
- *Be a Better Listener* by J.D. Obrice
- *The Compassion Method: Master Course,* a workbook by Laura Duncan
- *The Connection Codes* by Dr. Glenn and Phyllis Hill
- *I Hear You* by Michael S. Sorensen
- *Imperfect Parenting* by Brittney Serpell
- *Indestructible* by Blake K. Healy

- *The Naked Gospel* by Andrew Farley
- *Numb to Known* by Aaron Zint

Other References Given in This Book

- 10 Loneliest Countries— https://www.worldatlas.com/places/10-loneliest-nations-in-the-world.html
- Laura Duncan—https://www.lauraduncan.com
- Aaron and Jenna Zint—-www.zintsquad.com
- Lisa Kalfus—https//www.firestartconnections.com
- Brittney and Ben Serpell—www.lovingonpurpose.com
- Dr. Daniel Amen—https://danielamenmd.com
- Dr. Caroline Leaf—https://drleaf.com
- Francis Frangipane—https://frangipane.org
- Love McPherson—https://www.lovemcpherson.com
- Dr. Josh Axe—https://draxe.com
- Dr. Gabor Maté—https://drgabormate.com
- Tony Robbins—https://www.tonyrobbins.com
- Blake K. Healy—http://blakekhealy.com
- Dan and Nancy Barrett—https://www.untilnowcreative.org

Additional resources can be found at:

Leslie Parker Taylor—www.leslieparkertaylor.com

Email: leslieparkertaylor@gmail.com

ACKNOWLEDGMENTS

A sincere thank you:

To my husband, Tom Taylor, my safe place, the holder of my heart, who supports my ambitions, even at a cost to himself, and who loves me well all the time.

To my family—my sons, Kobey and Chase; my daughter-in-love, Jenni; and my grandkids, Madison, Kade, Reese, and Brienna. You are a gift. I love you so much.

To my favorite graphic artist, my brother Tommy G. Parker, who helped me on this project and many others over the years. I am so grateful and truly can't thank you enough.

To Linda Brooks, that special friend who is more like a sister. Thank you for believing in me, encouraging me, and even prodding me at times to write—for some thirty years. Thank you for not letting me forget what you felt I was called to do and for contributing to the process by reading every draft I sent you.

To my friend, Candyce Roberts, PhD in theology, who works in trauma recovery and inner healing prayer ministry (Candyce_lee_3@yahoo.com). Thank you for reading my rough draft and sharing your encouragement, author to author.

To my friend, Karen Hauck, owner/founder of Evexia Consulting (https://evexia.live). Thank you for reading my rough draft, sharing your thoughts, and giving input along the way.

To Linda, Candyce, and Karen, each mentioned above—three very special long-distance friends who looked over this material and contributed feedback. I am grateful for the time and love you gave to me in doing so. I love you so much and appreciate your sacrifice on my behalf.

To Lynda Lynch, such a good friend for so long, who believes in me and has always made me feel special and smart. Everyone needs a friend like Lynda.

To Connie Neuharth, my precious friend who continually covers me in prayer. I'm convinced her prayers have had a deep impact on my life and that I am alive today because of them.

To Kim Barry, Maryann Harper, and Christine Matthews—my three local BFFs, the ones who encircle me, who give me hugs whether they are needed or not, who always have an ear to give as I pour out my heart and process out loud, who

Acknowledgments

get excited for me in every adventure I undertake, who walk alongside me with an equal passion for Jesus, and who cover me in prayer continually.

To Jordan Pacilio, the original director and developer of Bethel Global Response, our local disaster team, for believing in me and giving me opportunities to teach and to grow. And to the entire BGR team, my local tribe, who have been the most awesome lovers of Jesus and of people. You have always encouraged me as a pastor, a teacher, and a person, and you keep the bar raised high.

To my co-workers at the Transformation Center, who run alongside me, loving on people, helping them connect to God, to themselves, and to others, who have always supported my entrepreneurial adventures, and as fellow authors have encouraged the writing of this book.

To the leadership at Bethel Church Redding (www.bethel.com), to our senior leader Bill Johnson and associate senior leader Kris Vallotton, and to the rest of the leadership team at the church and ministry school, who continually provide teaching that challenges me to pursue more of God and who keep the fires burning in this environment with passion for the Lord.

To Danny Silk, founder of Loving On Purpose (www.lovingonpurpose.com), a senior leader at Bethel Church Redding who hired me as director of Pastor on Call (POC) at Bethel back in 2009, opening the door to so many opportunities and relationships that have deeply impacted my life. Thank you, Danny, for also writing the foreword to this book.

To Chris Gore, Jason Vallotton, Dawna De Silva, Yvonne Martinez, and Janine Mason for writing endorsements. I truly can't thank you enough. Thank you for taking the time and for your kind words and support.

To Eric Johnson, now lead pastor at Studio in Greenville, South Carolina, who prophesied over me seventeen years ago that I would write two books. At the time, I remember being shocked, and then immediately thinking, "Only two?" But over the years, that word from the Lord through Eric has served as an anchor to my belief that I would eventually get there. I guess I am a good testimony for not giving up. I'm halfway there!

And proof that it truly takes a village to get a book written:

A special thanks to my mentor at selfpublishing.com, Brett Hilker, who gave me the tracks to run on and who helped me to go from a blank piece of paper to something I could call a manuscript to hand to an editor.

To my two editors, Nancy Pile and Christine Tracy. I am so indebted.

Acknowledgments

To my developmental editor, Nancy Pile (www.zoowrite.com), inspired editor, ghostwriter, and proofreader, who quickly captured my heart, kept me encouraged, and made me sound good. You have been such an incredible joy to work with. This book is so much better than it started out because of you.

To my dear friend, Christine Tracy (www.christinetracy.com), writing coach, blogger, and author of *Essence: 365 God Thoughts About You*, who graciously came on as a second editor. Thank you for initially reading my various drafts as a friend and then agreeing to jump on officially with the final manuscript. I love you bunches and so appreciate you making time for me. Your editing wisdom added just the right touches and made this book that much better.

And lastly, a big thank you to Nikki in Customer Service at Selfpublishing.com and the rest of the team. You got me to the finish line. Thank you!

I have known for a long time that I needed to write. I've had prophetic words that I should write. I've had encouragement to write from random people my entire life. I even had an encounter with the Lord in which He told me to stop editing and start writing, and another encounter in which He told me to stop being so hungry for what He was telling others (by reading) and start sharing what He was telling me (by writing). Even at that, I floundered. So when I came across Selfpublishing.com and saw they would give me tracks to run on and guidance all along the way, I knew that's what it would take to get my first book done. They say the first book is the hardest. I thought I picked an easy topic to start with, but boy, it has not been an easy process! I've written chapters in other books that were easy, but this is my first stand-alone book. I can only hope this is the hardest one and that it gets easier from here. At least I will have an idea of the process for the next one. Many thanks to everyone who has sown into me and encouraged me along the way!

ABOUT THE AUTHOR

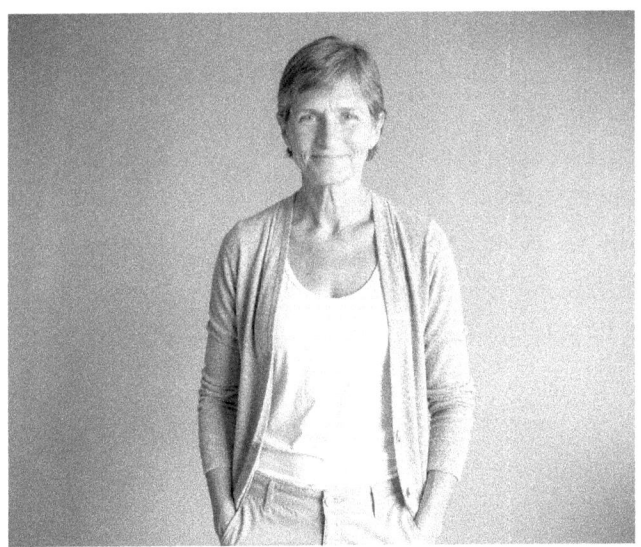

Leslie Taylor is a therapist offering individual and couples counseling at Bethel Church's Transformation Center in Redding, California. Many clients come to Leslie with burning questions like "Am I broken?" and "Am I weird?" And she helps give them a sense of what is and isn't normal in their life and relationships. Together, they brainstorm for solutions. Her clients continually express that working with Leslie makes them feel valued, seen, and heard, and they experience a fresh wave of hope, healing, and direction.

Leslie was born and raised in Stillwater, Oklahoma. She moved with her young family to Fort Collins, Colorado, where she lived for twenty-five years. She and her husband, Tom, later moved to Redding, California, where she attended ministry school.

Closest to Leslie's heart are her husband, her daughter in heaven, her two sons, her daughter-in-love, and her four grandchildren.

She loves many things, but a few of her favorites are a warm, sandy beach, jigsaw puzzles, riding her bike, watching the birds feeding in her backyard, easy hikes, and lunch dates with friends.

To learn more about Leslie or to contact her, go to www.leslieparkertaylor.com.

www.ingramcontent.com/pod-product-compliance
Lightning Source LLC
Chambersburg PA
CBHW060455030426
42337CB00015B/1604